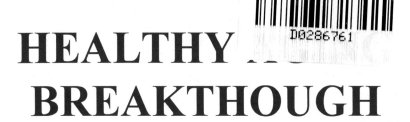

# HEALTHY
# BREAKTHOUGH

∞

## Amazing New Supplements, and diet for ideal Weight and Degenerative Disease Prevention

**Nicholas Delgado, M.S., Ph.D.**

**Health Wellness Studios, Inc.**
Lake Forest, California

**Proper Medical Care Suggestion & Disclaimer**
The ideas in this book are based on what the author would do if any disease conditions faced the author, what he would do to meet his needs. Nick is a health professional and is not claiming to be a licensed physician. The suggestions are based on the scientific information currently available, and you are encouraged to share this information with your doctor. If you are on medications you may need to adjust your dosages, so please consult your physician to monitor your progress and medical needs. We disclaim any liability arising from this book when you self medicate or take responsibility for your own care.

Health Wellness Studios Inc. books may be purchased for education use. For information to order single copies or multiple copy discounts write at:
25422 Trabuco Road, building 105, suite 141, Lake Forest, CA 92630
1-800-631-0232

First Edition

**Library of Congress Cataloging-in-Publication Data**
**98-94176**
**Delgado, Nick, 1955**

Healthy Aging Breakthrough: Amazing Supplements for Ideal Weight & Disease Prevention
Includes bibliographical references and index.
**ISBN 1-879084-05-8 (paper back)**   $15.95

Cover Designed by GEOS-Reprographics, Irvine California
Manufactured in the United States of America

# About The Author

**Nick Delgado, Author, Speaker and Radio Show Host**

Nicholas R. Delgado, Jr., Ph.D., is the Director of Healthy Studios Inc. After graduating from the University of Southern California (U.S.C.) with a BA degree in Psychology, he began his postgraduate studies in Physical Therapy at U.S.C. Rancho Los Amigos Hospital, followed by volunteer work at Daniel Freeman Hospital and Chino Hospital. Through his experiences in physical therapy, Nick Delgado became deeply concerned by the large numbers of people dying from such degenerative diseases as heart disease, stroke, diabetes and cancer.

Nick was motivated to undertake in-depth postgraduate studies in nutrition at Cal State Los Angeles and Cal State Long Beach University. He also spent years studying medical journals at U.S.C. and U.C. Irvine in his search for solutions to degenerative diseases. In 1982, Loma Linda University offered a Masters leading to a Doctorate program in Health Science and Delgado was accepted as a Doctoral candidate. Loma Linda School of Public Health was founded by Christians who followed the vegetarian type diet described in the bible that is free of meat and dairy products. They were motivated to do research based on holistic nutrition and exercise. Most universities in the country only offered dietitian training based on the outdated four foods group provided by the dairy and meat industry sponsored textbooks. In 1993, Nick was accepted to do independent research under academic guidance at the American Holistic College of Nutrition. Doctor Nick Delgado completed his Ph.D. thesis by doing a study on 693 people in a wellness program provided at seminars with Tony Robbins. Nick received his Ph.D. in Health Science.

He began to apply what he was learning to his medical problems of obesity and high blood pressure. After just five months Nick reduced 50 lb. of body fat, and lowered his blood pressure (from 200/90 to 110/70) and was able to get off blood pressure medications. Nick has maintained optimum health for over 20 years and at the age of 42 he competed in an intense strength and endurance test in Kona, Hawaii and set a record at that time against all participants of any age.

Nick then developed his highly successful nutrition, exercise, motivation and stress management program (forerunner to today's Healthy Aging Plan). In 1979, Nick became the Director of the Pritikin Better Health

Program studying with the famous research scientist, Nathan Pritikin. Nathan Pritikin taught Nick Delgado to sift through the misinformation and take complex medical journals and make it easy for everyone to understand them. Nick teamed up with health experts and looked for consistent themes of aging and disease and came up with new answers to these age-old problems. Nick Studied with Nathan Pritikin at the Longevity Center for three years, during this period he met and studied with many world-renowned scientists, including Denis Burkitt, MD, Ernest Wynder, MD, Arnold Fox MD, and Cleaves Bennett MD.

Later that year, Nick became involved with creating a wellness program centered in hospitals and with medical groups. In December, 1982, Nick began education and medical services in Southern California. Nick Delgado puts on dynamic seminars and refers to counseling services with anti-aging doctors and highly trained professionals. The Healthy Aging plan has enabled thousands of participants to feel better and become renewed. In all, Nick has presented over 20 years: 3,500 seminars at medical clinics, hospitals, community centers and large corporations including Aerospace and TRW. In 1992 to 1997 he set up and provided wellness testing using live blood cell hematology, oxidative stress analysis, carotid artery scans, blood lipids, biochemical hormones and seminars for over 10,000 participants with Tony Robbins Mastery University.

Nick is now considered one of the leading wellness advocates in the nation. In 1999, Nick began a national education program on talk radio CBS's KLSX 97.1 FM, and on KKLA 99.5 FM called Health & Wealth to share his incredible discoveries with those wanting more out of life. Nick has appeared on over 1,000 radio and TV talk shows. Nick did undergraduate work at the Academy of Fine Arts, USC, well know for turning out great producers, directors of media, and he completed studies in Psychology. His ability to answer live questions on the air with compassion, demonstrates his uncanny understanding of human needs, emotion and the will to survive and achieve. His charismatic personality, healthy appearance and contagious energy invites people to purse the healthy aging program with passion.

Surely you want to avoid the pain and suffering of the disease called aging? Wouldn't it be better to prevent premature aging and disease? You now can read the book "*Healthy Aging Breakthrough*", by Nick Delgado and learn the solutions to most conditions believed to be of unknown cause or aging. Why do most books only have part of the answers, missing the big picture and all the steps to getting to the cause of the problem? The answers have been lost in the tons of medical literature and confused by personal bias of studies sponsored by special interest groups like pharmaceutical companies, the meat, dairy, and processed food giants.

Is there a need for wellness care? Over 100 million Americans are in poor health with one or more chronic illness or degenerative diseases. One and one half billion prescriptions were written in 1997 or seven prescriptions for every single U.S. citizen. However, the fascinating fact is that over $6,000,000,000 (billion) was spent on vitamins, minerals, enzymes, herbs, homeopathic preparations, and amino acids. *Newsweek Magazine* predicted a phenomenal 20% rate of growth for supplement sales in just the U.S. One-third of Americans use alternative therapies, spending over $14 billion a year on unconventional treatments. People realize that a preventative approach to illness and an interest in enhanced vitality, energy level and longevity is possible with the Healthy Aging program.

Nick Delgado is the author and publisher of six books including his current book "*How to Look Great and Feel Sexy*", a cookbook that gives you the latest steps and 100's of tasty recipes (Italian, Chinese, Mexican, Thai and American cuisine's) on fat loss and nutrition. In his newest book, *Healthy Aging Breakthrough* and on his radio shows, or audio tapes, Nick will teach you about the best supplements, vitamins, minerals, enzymes, phytochemicals, biochemical hormones, herbs and nutrition to use for you and your family. Many of the complaints associated with aging such as obesity, sagging, wrinkled skin, loss of energy and libido, heart disease, cancer, arthritis, diabetes, bone loss and digestive problems can be alleviated or reduced with this healthy aging wellness plan.

The bible describes a healthy aging solution in Daniel "Please test your servants for ten days: Give us nothing but vegetables to eat and water to drink. Then compare our appearance with that of the young men who eat the royal food and wine. .... At the end of the ten days they looked healthier and better nourished than any of the young men who ate the royal food. So the guard took away their choice food and the wine they were to drink and gave them vegetables and water instead." Delgado and his associates have taken what is known in current medical science and put together a program with supplements and therapies that is practical, has tasty foods, and easy to follow.

To order Nick's Books, tapes, find out where to get supplements or therapy, radio or TV show appearances, or to schedule him as guest or keynote speaker call 888-517-7421 or for general information write to use and send a self address stamped envelope to Health Wellness Studios 25422 Trabuco Road # 105-141 Lake Forest CA 92630, or call 800-631-0232.

# Table of Contents

# Acknowledgements

This book represents over 20 years of searching for the truth about our bodies and how to live life at its' best. I want to thank all of those individuals who like me have found new answers and were willing to share them with me in their interviews, writings, seminars, and influences. They were not always the richest, or the loudest. I do believe they were the best at coming up with practical solutions and better systems to living a quality life. Nathan Pritikin, John McDougall MD, Tony Robbins, Bob Wieland, Shawna Kendell, Dr. Barbara Brewitt, Michael Klaper M.D., John Robbins, Wayne Dyer, Zig Ziglar, Dennis Estabrook, Brian Sutton, David Steenblock DO., Theresa Crenshaw MD., Jonathan Wright M.D., John Lee M.D., Dr. William Timmins, Arnold Fox MD.

Thank you

# INTRODUCTION

This book combines the collective experiences of the Healthy Aging staff in helping people like yourself. Perhaps you have a health problem, or maybe you would like to experience optimum health. Read this book, start exercising, and begin the nutrition plan, experience the amazing power of supplements and biochemical replacements and you can benefit or improve in the following areas:

In the first section of this book, we will review the three hormonal systems that decline with age; According to: *Science Vol. 278, Oct 1997,*

1. **Somatopause-** occurs when men and women age because of a decrease in human growth hormone released by the pituitary gland causing a decrease in the production of Insulin Like Growth factor (IGF-1) by the liver and other organs.

2. **Menopause - in women** happens when follicle-stimulating hormone (FSH) decreases, reducing the secretion of estrogen & progesterone.
   **Andropause - in men** happens when gonadotropin luteinizing hormone (LH) decreases, reducing secretion of testosterone.

3. **Adrenopause – DHEA** production decreases in both men and women as adrenocortical cells produce less DHEA.

What if we replace these hormones by using natural supplements identical to our body's hormone molecules or by stimulating the production of hormones with precursor stimulants and herbs to stop suppression or blocking, allowing the release of these hormone levels to more youthful levels. WE CAN SLOW or REVERSE AGING!

This **Healthy Aging** plan has been written about in thousands of journals, and witnessed by over 5,000 physicians in clinical practices world-wide. We will share with you what 30 years of research has discovered about the aging process. We give you a simple system for you to improve your diet using the exciting and amazingly easy **blending** of vegetables and fruit, carrying a **Cool tote** filled with your favorite nibbler foods, and the **Supplement Box.** You will learn about how to pick and choose the best supplements, herbs, enzymes, and biochemical enhancers. You will learn how to identify allergies, increase energy, fat loss methods, and exercise for busy people.

In the second part of this book you will learn how to prevent the ravages of degenerative disease by identifying the cause and the steps to prevention:

The Healthy Aging staff would like you to live a longer, healthier, happier life. Living a longer, healthier life is important to you and your family, isn't it? And yet, there is a myth about life expectancy in the United States. Because of our lower infant mortality rate, people mistakenly think we're healthier; however, past the age of 40, we rank 38th in the world in life expectancy in a recent study comparing 60 nations! Though our country has the best of medical technology, you still have a greater chance than ever before of dying prematurely from atherosclerosis, heart disease, cancer, diabetes or hypertension. In fact, 1 1/2 million people die every year from these causes alone.

If you were to drop dead suddenly from heart disease without any debilitating symptoms, that might not be so bad. But it doesn't usually work that way. Most people in their last 20 years of life slowly lose functions - hearing, sight, etc. Their joints ache, blood pressure rises, there are side effects from medications, sexual impotency occurs and they lose their zest for life. If you could discover how to reduce or prevent these and other serious illnesses - how to achieve the ideal level of health, and significantly extend your life - you would, wouldn't you? The Healthy Aging Plan is now available to you as a complete educational, motivational and personalized approach. It can help you and your family to improve the quality of life.

Comparing your health to people in optimum or ideal health provides helpful insight. There are over 800 million people on the Healthy Aging Plan type of diet: high in complex carbohydrates and fiber, low in fat and cholesterol. In these countries (25 populations examined) we find almost no killer diseases such as heart disease, and they have a longer life expectancy past the age of 40. In contrast, one out of every three adults in this country is suffering from cardiovascular disease. What is wrong with the American diet?

Is your diet high in fat? Do you know that cheddar cheese and peanut butter are 71% fat? Margarine, corn oil and butter 100% fat and sirloin steak is 77% fat? The average American also eats many hidden fats, because processed sugars also turn into fat. This can cause your bloodstream to become clogged with fats, resulting in poor circulation.

**OBESITY, WEIGHT LOSS OR GAIN, IDEAL WEIGHT** - This book will teach you how to improve nutrition with water rich foods and exercise to reduce the size of your fat cells to ideal level. You will also discover the surprising reason why declining hormone levels cause you to gain fat. The special supplements you need will correct this problem and build muscle instead of fat. Could it be that the fast foods, TV dinners and high levels of sugar, fat, cholesterol and salt that we were raised on lead to illness and heart disease? Combine these with a lack of exercise, obesity or smoking, processed foods devoid of essential nutrients and declining biochemical hormone levels and your risk for developing heart disease climbs even higher.

Heart disease is gradual. The average closure of the 20-year-old's coronary arteries is already 20%. The average closure of a 35-year-old is almost 50%. When you are 45 years of age, you may have a 90% closure and it's at this late stage that you'll have your first symptom: angina (chest pain). If your arteries to the brain narrow, you may have signs of dizziness, headaches, senility or even stroke.

The tragedy is that most people with so-called "average" cholesterol levels of 160 to 240 have hardening (narrowing) of the arteries. If you're smart, you'll want to prevent further damage to your arteries. The Healthy Aging Plan can help you do this by bringing your cholesterol level down to safer levels. Dr. W. Castelli, cardiologist, has stated that "diet could reverse (dissolve) coronary artery disease plaques in 90% of the patients if we got everyone's cholesterol below 150 mg."

**HEART DISEASE & HARDENING OF THE ARTERIES:** Most of the known factors that lead to artery closures will be lowered or eliminated. Your blood cholesterol level may drop an average of 20% (the harmful LDL will come down the most, while the good HDL stabilizes). You can reduce or eliminate medications for heart disease, angina, hypertension, diabetes and obesity with the assistance of this book and the monitoring of your health professional.

**CANCER** - Cancer is the second major cause of death in the U.S. The National Cancer Institute and the American Cancer Society now fully support the contention that cancer is in large part preventable, and if it should develop, there is new evidence to show that cancer of the breast, prostate, colon and uterus is treatable. Research on a low-fat, zero cholesterol, high-fiber Healthy aging diet has shown exciting results in the fight against cancer. These same foods help the blood to be slightly alkaline which can retard tumor growth. Biochemical hormone balance also enhances the immune system to protect and rebuild the body.

**PROSTATE DISORDERS, MALE SEXUAL IMPOTENCE** - Can be helped through proper medical management using various solutions based on your specific needs. An alarming number of men develop prostate cancer. Evidence shows that maintaining a low cholesterol level could prevent cancer cases. Avoiding the accumulation of cholesterol is of critical importance to the health of the prostate gland. A high cholesterol level is now considered a leading cause of sexual impotence due to clogged arteries and restricted blood flow to the penis. Amazing herbs and supplements restore youthful hormone levels and potency.

**HIGH BLOOD PRESSURE (HYPERTENSION)** - By following the six effective steps to controlling blood pressure as outlined in this book, you may free yourself of the need for medications in just twelve weeks. Without our comprehensive system, most people fail because they usually just reduce salt and use medications. By contrast, we teach you the steps to reducing fat in your circulation that frees your body of stress. The supplements we use help restore the elasticity of the arteries.

**DIABETES, HYPOGLYCEMIA** - The Healthy Aging Plan has generated considerable excitement within the medical community through its success in helping people to reach their ideal blood sugar levels in as little as eight weeks using the water rich complex carbohydrates and reduced fat in your diet. The American Diabetic Association has found that a Healthy Aging-type approach can successfully help most diabetics to reduce their need for insulin dramatically. According to Dr. Kelly West, endocrinologist, and Dr. James Anderson, 62% of adult onset diabetics could get off insulin and other drugs, and return to ideal health in less than three months.

**GLAUCOMA, CATARACTS, EYESIGHT** - There are people in the world who rarely develop these eye disorders so common in our culture. Medical research shows that excess fat in the bloodstream can lead to a pressure buildup in the eye, damaging the retina (nerves in the eye) that can cause the progressive loss of eyesight. The Healthy Aging Plan can reduce the intraocular pressure in the eye and prevent the need for eye drops. Many cases of cataracts are related to high cholesterol levels, eye drops for glaucoma and impurities (sorbitol), which ruin the clarity of the lens. You can look forward to a life virtually free of these eye disorders by following our program.

Like most people, you probably don't have the endurance capabilities of the famous Tarahumara Indians in Northern Mexico, who run nonstop for 48 hours - a distance of 175 miles! They are free of degenerative diseases because they eat a healthy diet and exercise regularly. Their blood relatives, though, the Pima Indians in Phoenix, eat a high fat diet, and as a result have a very high rate of arthritis, diabetes and gallstones.

**ARTHRITIS:** As you learn to improve your circulation, you can reduce the pain and stiffness in your joints. Allergies with elimination of specific foods combined with supplements can slow degeneration in your spine, knees, fingers, shoulders and feet.

**ASTHMA & EMPHYSEMA** - As your lung capacity improves through our program of mild aerobic exercises, improved nutrition to reduce fatty blood, allergy identification with specific food elimination and smoking cessation assistance; everyone experiences enhanced breathing capabilities.

**CONSTIPATION-HEMORRHOIDS, COLITIS, DIVERTICULOSIS, ULCERS, VARICOSE VEINS AND GALLSTONES:** -These digestive disorders can be prevented, or, if present, often relieved by following the Healthy Aging plan because of the use of natural fibers and exercise to stimulate and properly soothe the digestive tract.

**KIDNEY & LIVER DISORDERS** - A high protein diet, alcohol and fat inhibit the function and damage these vital organs. The Healthy Aging Plan offers amazing new biochemical hormone supplements to restore organ size.

**MENSTRUAL DISORDERS (PMS), MENOPAUSE** - The use of the Healthy Aging Plan for female hormone imbalances is safe and effective without the need for drugs. Daily exercise and a low-fat diet are the cornerstone therapies combined with natural hormone replacement supplements without drugs.

**OSTEOPOROSIS** - You can start rebuilding your bones with exercise, supplements, and reduced protein (non-acidic) foods. Natural progesterone cream will prevent the loss of bone material.

We at the Healthy Aging Plan believe that whole natural foods, low in fat, low in cholesterol, along with sensible supplementation, are your best medicine. Exercise, a positive attitude, and a spiritual commitment will provide the most comprehensive known program leading you on the path to good health. We can refer you to medical doctors and health educators who are dedicated to helping you achieve your goals following the Healthy Aging Plan.

For more information, to order cassette tapes on the exciting information covered in this book, or to make an appointment at a referral clinic for a Healthy Aging, Please call us at (800) 631-0232.

*I have spent over twenty years studying aging, nutrition, exercise, physiology, and reviewing medical research. I reviewed over 250,000 reports and lectured with Nathan Pritikin of the Pritikin Longevity Center. I conducted tests on over 10,000 participants at Mastery University events with Tony Robbins. I believe that you can remain physically and emotionally strong with advanced age.*

*We have all heard about the need to consume healthy foods and supplements. We know about the benefits of exercise. My experience as a seminar speaker, TV and radio talk show host, shows me that only about 10% of the people follow a good lifestyle plan. Some people are confused and they make the excuse they do not have the time or money necessary to do independent research to know which is the best program for them. How can we help the other 90% that are in need of help and how can we improve the performance of the 10% interested in outstanding results? People want a simplified and practical program that I call the "Healthy Aging Plan".*

# I

∞

# Natural Breakthrough for the Disease called Aging

**Man age 74 turns the clock back looks 40!**

What if you could live to age 100 in as healthy and as vigorous a condition as you were when you were age 25? Is it possible? Can we help you turn the clock back? I would like to share with you the example of a man age 74, named Bob. He read an article in Longevity magazine and decided to replace his biochemical levels to achieve the fountain of youth. He is a California bodybuilder and after a six-month period of human growth hormone ( or GH) replacement, he looked like a man of age 40 in great shape! Everyone past the age of 30 begins the process of aging: sagging wrinkled thin skin, increased body fat, sagging breasts, sagging abdomen, pot belly, thin hair and fatigue. The aging clock starts because our biochemical hormones levels are decreasing.

**HGH -The Fountain of Youth?**

We have identified the 8 critical hormones that decline with age; the most important one of them is the master hormone known as human growth hormone (HGH). Growth is somewhat of a misnomer. It is called growth because it is so critical during that phase of growth of all children. A better name would have been rejuvenation hormone or possibly the fountain of youth hormone. As evidence, past the age of forty, if we restore this hormone we can see some rather amazing results in people reversing the signs of aging.

Up until recently the way to administer HGH was through **injection**. A few years back as my levels started to decline I decided to undergo HGH injection therapy. I did this for a six-month period under the guidance of three different doctors. I am a researcher and I have studied with some of the top doctors in the country who work with anti-aging therapy. Neal Rouzier MD, Foud Ghaly MD, and Jack Palmer MD have treated over 50 physicians, all of whom were initially skeptical of this new therapy. It is not until one tries this new therapy and experiences the tremendous increased vigor that one realizes the harm that is being caused to the body by the lack of these hormones.

During this six-month period I found a tremendous restoration of my health and fitness levels. However, I was a little discouraged with the cost of this type of therapy. The cost runs somewhere around $1200 per month or more and you also have to deal with injections once or twice a day. Most people I talked to felt that even though the therapy sounded valid and worthwhile they would not want to subject themselves to daily injections, let alone the cost involved. So that led me to a search of alternatives that could be utilized...natural replacements. I came across a natural oral replacement for HGH.

Being rather curious, I had my baseline IGF-1 (Insulin Like Growth Factor) level measured before I began any type of oral therapy. The highest measurement of my IGF-1 on injectables were never above 241 ng/ml and after going off of injectables my levels declined down to between 174 ng/ml and 195 ng/ml. Those levels may be consistent with a man of age 41, but they were unacceptable based on youthful goals. So I began using the **oral replacement** for HGH and within eight weeks my repeat blood tests revealed my IGF-1 levels had climbed to 349 ng/ml. This was a level you would find in a 25-year-old! I noticed the same very similar exciting results that I had encountered using injection. Physically I noticed increase in strength, increase in muscle density and an improvement in sexual prowess in the bedroom. I was extremely happy to know that I could receive the same results as the injections with the oral replacement. When you look at these kinds of results you have to wonder why more doctors haven't used this simple healthy aging therapy.

Since hormones decline in all people as they age it's easy to see why so many physicians assume this is natural. However, if a younger person were to be diagnosed with a hormonal deficiency, this would quickly be corrected. Unfortunately, physicians have not been trained to treat middle-aged people with a deficiency if it's believed to be associated with aging. Researchers around the world have shown hormonal deficiency at any age, young or old, require replacement. If you decide to correct your hormones, do it under a doctor's guidance. If you take supplements on your own, without testing, you are self-diagnosing and must assume your own risk.

**HGH** is the master hormone. So when I decided to start taking the oral HGH replacement, I stopped taking all the other natural replacements such as DHEA, melatonin or herbs for testosterone even though I had been measured to be low in these biochemical levels. I wanted to get the feel for what HGH by itself would do for me. I was happy to see all the great results from oral HGH that I reported earlier using injectables. Once I had proven to myself that I had improved physically after two months I re-tested my blood levels at 349 ng/ml. I continued using natural oral HGH for a full six months. Then I resumed taking low dosages of DHEA, Melatonin, and testosterone stimulating herbs since these biochemical hormones work together synergistically with HGH.

### Lose Fat by replacing hormones

So I ask you this question, how many of you would like to achieve your ideal weight? Weight control has become more of a problem, especially past the age of 40. Eighty percent of the weight gain has been identified as a result of the change of hormones! So if we could correct the hormones, we could actually help people to get to their ideal body weight.

### Low fat diet & exercise kept me fit when I was under age 40

I look back to my own situation where I at one time was quite obese (over 210 pounds), and at over 35% body fat. I struggled with obesity throughout childhood as a teenager and into adulthood. There were brief periods when I was able to lose the weight during athletics while following starvation type diets. Unfortunately, as I ate the typical western diet high in fat, meat and dairy products, I gained more and more weight. It was really exciting for me to learn that through a change in diet and exercise, I was able to lose 40 to 50 pounds of body fat and was able to keep it off for years.

17

## Hormone therapy-a must after 35 years old

However, as I got older, I noticed the decline in hormone levels, even though I was doing the same strict diet and exercise and keeping on track. It was difficult to keep my weight down and energy up. It wasn't until I started the hormone therapies and monitored my levels that I began to notice that I needed fewer workouts. I didn't have to go to the gym two times a day to keep up with my younger years. In fact, I was able to only go to the gym about three to five times a week like it was when I was in my twenties. I did increase my muscle density quite considerably and I noticed a weight gain of nearly 8 pounds of lean muscle mass and a drop in body fat. In my case there was not a change in body weight overall because I had gained muscle and lost fat.

## HGH reduces body fat & restores protein

HGH has also been shown to reduce fat because it actually helps fat to be utilized for energy and it conserves the carbohydrates. HGH also increases the rate at which the protein is utilized in the cells to restore cells and organs to youthful levels.

### Improved fluid balance

As we age, we dehydrate and actually begin to dry up. Our bodies, muscles and organs are made up of over 70% water. HGH and human growth factors (IGF-1) restore low levels of extracellular fluid. By replenishing this water, I noticed my skin became thicker and wrinkles became less noticeable. Also, I noticed an improvement in perspiration capacity during exercise. The HGH and growth factors also normalize kidney function.

### How to increase your energy

How many of you reading this would like to have more energy? Now if you can barely respond I know you need more energy! Most adults struggle through life with fatigue. Somewhere past the age of 20 or 25 that energy level declines. And what is it? Is it all just a change in eating habits, not enough sleep, or lack of exercise? The decline in energy is not just lifestyle; it is related to a decline in biochemical hormone levels involved with the aging process. When you restore the levels of HGH, DHEA, testosterone, progesterone, and thyroid, your energy levels start to be restored as well. I know my energy levels have improved tremendously.

**First improve your diet & exercise for peak performance**

I put Shawna Kendell, my associate and partner, on a peak performance diet called the Healthy Aging Diet by increasing raw food using a whole food blender; blending vegetables, sprouts and fruit drink every morning. She began eating frequent small meals of salads, fruit and vegetarian food prepared low in fat. She started weight training combined with aerobic exercise. Within a few months she had made tremendous progress and reported feeling better than she had in years.

**Step two is add vitamins & minerals and enzymes**

We analyzed a sample of blood checking for acidic blood, free radical damage, and vitamin or mineral deficiencies. We looked at her prior test results and did further checks for anemia. We also did lipid panels and looked for excess fat circulating in the blood known as triglycerides. The shape and quality of her red blood cells looked great. However, the level of fat in her blood was too high, even though she appeared to be at a good body weight. After eating the suggested frequent meals low in fat, her circulation improved within days and she began feeling better.

**Hormone levels past age 30 are low & need replacement**

Next we referred her to an anti-aging doctor that was willing to measure her blood and saliva for the 8 critical hormones. Shawna was low in thyroid, DHEA, estrogen, Free Testosterone and HGH (HGH). She shared information at a recent seminar about her changes in energy as we changed her diet, exercise, added supplements and restored her biochemical hormone levels. "I had been seeing a physician for a couple of years. They were looking for things such as chronic fatigue syndrome and lupus. After extensive testing they told me they could find nothing physically wrong with me and wanted to prescribe antidepressants. It was after that point, I started with Nick's Healthy Aging wellness program combined with hormone therapy."

**Restore energy by wellness program & HGH**

"I am so glad I decided to try an alternate route of wellness taught by Nick Delgado. The medical doctor Nick referred me to suggest that I have my biochemical levels checked and I was surprised to find out that several of my levels were quite low. I started taking natural replacements for HGH. My energy increased tremendously. I would wake up in the morning feeling refreshed and that energy continued through the entire day. It was a lifesaver for me. I am the mother of 5 children ages 9 to 20 so to keep up with all of them and all their activities is very important to me."

## Oral homeopathic HGH works best

Shawna had obtained these great results using the oral replacement for HGH. Her baseline IGF-1 level started at 221 ng/ml and after 8 weeks of consistent use of the oral replacement, her IGF-1 levels jumped to 424 ng/ml. That is the level of a 20-year-old! Needless to say she was excited to find how simple it was to achieve that level. People around her were noticing the change in her skin texture, muscle tone and her appearance. Shawna at age 37 looks very young and is in great shape.

I remember her calling me after a few months because she had ran out of the product. She had been out for about 2 weeks and was noticing the change. She had not fully realized how beneficial the product was for her until she was without it. Since she has been back on HGH, she has seen a reduction in cellulite that she was never able to get rid of with exercise. Her mental clarity has improved. Her muscles have become toned and firm and she has increased endurance in the gym and in life in general.

We made certain that HGH was the only thing she took after we established her baseline with the best possible diet and exercise program. Once Shawna obtained the benefits of HGH, we then encouraged her to replace her other deficient hormones for DHEA, thyroid, melatonin, testosterone, estrogen, and progesterone. Shawna noticed additional improvements in how she looked and felt. Her outlook on life regarding health is one of complete confidence regarding healthy aging.

Shawna noticed similar results as I did. Her weight went up about 4 pounds but her body fat dropped from 28% down to 20%. She remarked that the thing that she noticed the very most was that her body could once again do the things her mind still thought it could do like when she was younger. Our results are indicators of what we consider a reversal in aging. We did nothing different in our eating habits or exercise routine to help maintain our ideal weight. We found out how simple and easy it was to gain that lean body mass and reduce body fat. We follow a low-fat diet, high in water content, rich in vegetables, sprouts, and fruit, along with herbs, vitamins, and minerals. We have experienced the rejuvenate powers of biochemical hormones and supplements to achieve youthful levels.

Most people have a belief that we can wait until we get very old and then we can start doing intervention. We can find out what your hormone levels are and try to correct them at that point. However, by that time you have missed a critical period in your life. Why not consider aging gracefully? Why not do what we say in the medical community and that is to under go what we call "healthy aging"? **Healthy Aging** is something that wasn't available to us less than 18 years ago but now that the research is complete we can accomplish that.

### Myths about human longevity

There are examples of people in the world who have lived past 100 years of age, like the Hunza's of Pakistan. However, what you have to understand is that when we look at these reports very closely, these people have not lived as long as we have been led to believe. Some of what was reported in the medical journals showed that to avoid being inducted into the war the fathers passed their birth certificates on to their sons and it appeared that they were twice as old as they actually were. For example an individual age 70 was reported to be age 140. Yet this was not the case at all. So what really is the upper limits of life span? Somewhere between the ages of 120 to 125 is about accurate in terms of recorded length of man. Can we lengthen that or more importantly can we improve the quality of life up to that point? That is really the critical question that we have to ask.

Adults with low IGF-1 levels under 350 ng/ml have HGH (HGH) deficiency and can choose therapy or supplements, according to the FDA clearance given in 1986. Our levels HGH are highest during adolescence and decline rapidly past the age of 21. The pituitary gland produces HGH from pituitary cells called somatotrophs. Most HGH secretions occur in brief bursts, or pulses during the early hours of deepest sleep (Stage 4 of REM). Quality sleep is necessary to produce sufficient amounts of HGH. A 20-year-old produces 500 micrograms of HGH per day. A 40-year-old produces only 200 micrograms, and an 80-year-old produces barely 25 micrograms per day! Unfortunately as we age the length and quality of sleep declines and our bodies aren't able to rejuvenate. HGH pulses during sleep into the bloodstream and lingers for a few minutes until it reaches the liver and stimulates the production of growth factors such as IGF. IGF-1 or Insulin-like growth factor 1, also known as somatomedin C is responsible for most of the positive benefits of HGH.

The hypothalamus gland located in the brain monitors our body's HGH levels. This gland stimulates increased HGH levels by secreting GHRH (*human growth hormone releasing hormone*). If too much HGH is produced or the body perceives an excessive rise in insulin like growth factor IGF1, the hypothalamus gland can suppress pituitary output of HGH by secreting somatostain. *Somatostatin* shuts down the natural production of HGH until the levels drop back down in the system. As we get older, an excess increase in somatostain can cause premature aging.

There are **supplements** such as the amino acid L-arginine and Revostatin that help block excess somatostain. This can help to slow the aging process. Supplements that contain HGH, and insulin like growth factor IGF1 (to increase production of growth hormones and growth factor) can be taken with secretogogues like L-Glutamine (to increase hormonal secretion or release), along with revostatin or L-arginine (somatostain suppressors) to help restore our bodies to youthful levels.

The HGH *stimulates* the production of insulin like growth factor IGF-1 in the liver. IGF-1 then enhances the production of **albumin blood protein**. Albumin is essential for cell growth and renewal, regulates water balance to maintain hydration of cells, organs and transports nutrients such as amino acids to cells and removes waste from cells. It assists in the digestion of food, transports and buffers excess levels of all hormones, stabilizes blood pH so it's slightly alkaline and not too acidic, and serves as the ultimate antioxidant. Albumin maintains homeostasis or balance of the entire body.

I started reviewing the results that were available through other doctors using the natural oral homeopathic therapy. It was difficult to find doctors using the oral therapy because many of them were stuck on the idea that the only way to get good results was through injection. I tried to find why these doctors were so reluctant to try this very simple easy therapy. Some of the doctors I worked with began to decide that perhaps they could alternate therapy between oral replacement and injection to help reduce the cost of replacement therapy and thereby benefit the patient. I proposed that they put the patients on oral replacement only and then compare.

## Doctors test people using oral HGH

According to an unreported study on 60,000 people during a 6 year period (1989-1996) that cost over 2 million dollars by Dr. Robert Lawrence Ph.D., people using oral HGH showed an average increase of IGF-1 of 30%. I personally interviewed with a small group of doctors who were willing to test oral HGH. The typical patient was age 37 to 74, an equal group of male and female patients. The typical diagnose when they came in to see the doctor, included fatigue, depression, loss of sex drive and hyperthyroidism. These individuals had a baseline test for IGF-1 as well. They were re-tested within two to six months following their initial therapies. The average change in the first eleven patients that I reviewed went from 139 ng/ml to 202 ng/ml, for an average improvement of nearly 40%. The best improvements went from 199 to 282.

Shawna and I actually exceeded the results of the patients in this study with a 100% improvement in IGF-1 using oral homeopathic replacements. We were very consistent about using the oral HGH at least three times a day, morning, midday and evening. I went on to check another fourteen patients who had also done baseline tests with their doctor. They also showed remarkable results in how they felt including restored energy, improvement of libido, and a feeling of well being. As we look at the evidence and the research, we all have to take a very careful note of the results…and those results show a true reversal of the symptoms associated with aging.

## Oral-homeopathic-HGH restores body balance

In the mid 1980's companies started producing HGH through recombinant DNA technology. Special DNA is inserted into the DNA of microorganisms like yeast or friendly bacteria, causing the organism to reproduce a large supply of the identical 191 amino acid molecular make-up of our bodies' own HGH. In the early 1990's a scientist formerly with the NIH (National Institutes of Health), Barbara Brewitt, Ph.D., developed a patented homeopathic HGH product, in which actual recombinant HGH was used. Homeopathy is natural medicine based on the Law of Similars or "let like be cured by likes" which means like substances of very low dosages can be introduced into the body to stimulate the production and release of like substances, causing healing responses. By combining modern biotechnology, molecular biology and homeopathic principals, an alternative method of HGH delivery became available.

### Power of oral homeopathic growth factors

In 1995, Dr. Barbara Brewitt at University Health clinic in Washington and Dr. Leanna Standish, N.D, Ph.D., Director of Research at Bastyr University of Naturopathic Medicine did a four-month double-blind placebo-controlled clinical study to measure the power of homeopathic growth factors to enhance the immune system. Twenty-one patients with depressed immune systems or high viral activity and associated fatigue were tested. None of the patients were subjected to conventional antiviral drugs. One group was given only homeopathic oral growth factors with natural supplements of herbs, vitamins and minerals. The comparison placebo group was given the natural supplements of herbs, vitamins and minerals without homeopathic growth factors. Later the study included a crossover where the placebo group later was given the actual growth factors. Replication of the double-blind placebo controlled study occurred in seven different cities around the country on another 56 immune depressed patients. Research continued on a group of the patients for another two and one half years.

All clinical studies performed by Dr. Brewitt on the oral homeopathic products (human growth factors), were based on the standards of the *"Institutional Review Board"* composed of independent medical and scientific professionals associated with universities and medical treatment facilities.

### Amazing Results

The results of all of these clinical studies showed that oral administration of homeopathic growth factors strengthened the immune system and enhanced metabolism to fight viral activity as compared to placebo. People taking the homeopathic growth factors (including IGF1) gained up to 10 pounds of needed weight including muscle mass with one-third of them reaching ideal body weight. They had reduced rate of infection, lessened viral activity, improved T4 white cell counts, reduced inflammation throughout the body based on Sedimentation rates, improved mineral metabolism (especially calcium and phosphorus retention), all without side-effects. The placebo groups taking only herbs, vitamins and minerals without the homeopathic growth factors; experienced increased infections and viral activity, decreased T4 counts, and loss of weight, especially of lean muscle mass. These homeopathic growth factors (Cell Signal Enhancers®) enhance communication between your bodies' cells and cause better uptake of nutrients, which is very important to immune health and physical strength.

**Oral homeopathic HGH, studies: many benefits**      Dr. Brewitt went on to test the physiological effects of homeopathic HGH with healthy people ages 18 to 54 years old in a one month double-blind placebo controlled study. She wanted to see if oral administration of homeopathic HGH could have positive effects on healthy people just like the higher concentrations of injectable HGH. This was the first time a clinical study showed that homeopathic growth hormone taken orally could cause measurable effects in the blood stream. While the placebo group had no changes in their blood IGF1 levels, the group chewing a tablet of homeopathic HGH and allowed to absorb in their mouth had an 18 to 40% increase in blood IGF1 levels within two to four weeks! Additionally, Dr. Brewitt measured T4 white blood cell counts and found the immune systems of the people on treatment became stronger in measurable ways. People taking the oral homeopathic HGH gained lean **muscle mass**, felt **stronger** and more powerful with a greater enthusiasm for life and increased mental **clarity**.

**Depression elimination of with homeopathic growth factor**
    Dr. Brewitt has also conducted two different very small clinical studies on homeopathic IGF1 to evaluate how this molecule effects the nervous system. Insulin like growth factor IGF-1 is found all over the body, including the nervous system where it acts like a neuropeptide. In her clinical trials, she studied people who were healthy, but were psychologically depressed. The homeopathic IGF1 treatment surprised the psychotherapists who were seeing these people because these people felt better rapidly and measurably decreased or eliminated their depression after several months on treatments compared to placebo.

    Dr. Samuel Hahnemann, the 19th-century founder of homeopathy realized that remedies in large dosages almost always create negative side

25

effects. However, the same substance delivered in highly diluted minute doses, provided relief with no side effects. It has been often said, "Homeopathy is one of the rare medical approaches which carries no penalties-only benefits." Homeopathy is most effective using one remedy at a time to stimulate the person's natural defense system and raise the general level of health.

A product such as Homeopathic growth factor has actual Insulin like growth factor -1 potentization of 30C. Which means it has been diluted 30 times in one part active substance dissolved into 99 parts of water (Centesimal represents the "C" or 99 parts to 1). Therefore, the diluted medicine has been diluted again and again 30 times to reach the desired potency. For example, our bodies only manufacture up to 100 millionths of a gram of thyroid per day to regulate the entire body of a 200 lb. Person! That is just 1 part free thyroid per 10,000 million parts of blood plasma. Human growth factor that has been diluted more- is more powerful than the lower potencies, and should be used judiciously and according to the labeled use of three times a day.

**Discovery how homeopathic low dosage works**
Some doctors questioned how such small dosages that are used in homeopathy could get such powerful and effective results. Until physicists Liu, Cruzan, and Saykally at the University of California published a paper in the journal *Science, February 1996, Volume 271*, explaining how water could cluster in very specific networks. The networks formed around the originally diluted substances and formed crystalline mirror images, sometimes called (IE)"icy" crystals. Therefore, as homeopaths have said before, the networks and IE crystals retain their shape even after the original diluted substances (molecules of HGH) have vanished! It is theorized that these crystals in the homeopathic preparation of Cell Signal Enhancers® growth factors balance electromagnetic forces in the body, normalizing body system function. These growth factors, when prepared homeopathically make communications between cells possible sending signals and setting in motion the way cells use DNA. This stimulates the body's defenses, healing, and growth repair processes.

New cells are replacing dying cells in our body every minute at the rate of over 300 million replications! Communication between cells via growth factors to regulate and repair DNA before the cells next replication is critical to the healing process. Taste buds replace themselves every two weeks. The skin replaces every four weeks. The liver is renewed every six weeks. Your bones are completely replaced every year. Nearly 98% of all of our bodies' one hundred trillion living cells are replaced every year with new cells. If there is damage in the DNA coding, then this same defect will continue to replicate. In the case of arthritis, the same crippled joint is replaced with unhealthy tissue. The science of homeopathy, using actual **human growth factors**, stimulates the correction, repair and healing of the DNA feedback system. This actually allows the body to heal itself at the origin of the problem.

**Growth factors** such as homeopathic IGF-1 chewable tablets absorb in the mouth (sublingual) and balance the electromagnetic field with low dosage signals. This energy field is based on the same principal we've learned about when using acupuncture points for healing the body. This is an awesome and wondrous way to enhance the nervous system, immune system, hormone system and all other systems of the body. Add in raw enzyme rich food with herbs, supplements, daylight, exercise, fresh air and water to restore healthy cells.

Growth factors were found in the 1960's and by the 1980's we began to realize how important these little protein molecules are. Growth factors are messenger hormones that work within minutes of their presence to help cells talk to each other. Even if cells are right next to each other, the growth factors regulate the regeneration, growth and the aging of cells. Growth factors tell a cell when to live, when to die and when to specialize and perform only certain functions for the body. Without these growth factors we would become very ill. As we age, cells slow down and we need growth factors to awaken them to a more active phase.

The product with Growth factors (a class of over 40 very small proteins called polypeptides), including IGF-1 helps enhance mental clarity, endurance, reduction of pain, inflammation, fever, PMS and menopause symptoms. Many researchers and bodybuilders believe that IGF-1 is going to be as important a supplement as HGH has proven to be for looking and feeling younger.

The homeopathic product contains the actual recombinant HGH to assist in lean body mass and muscle strength as reported by athletes, and improvements in energy, endurance, and boosting the immune system.

The delivery of HGH and human growth factors orally includes taking the recombinant produced identical 191 amino acid molecule and preparing it homeopathically in the proper dilutions. This preserves the skeleton shape of the HGH as it passes through the filters of the mouth's mucous. We know absorption of the oral HGH is taking place because the IGF-1 levels increase significantly after daily use.

Other researchers have discovered the possibility of delivery by using polymer matrix to allow preservation and passage into the body. Water molecules, like other molecules (including HGH) have been found to be somewhat flexible and distortable. This may explain the way large molecules are able to pass thorough smaller membrane passageways. Pharmaceutical companies have begun using liposomal technology to deliver many different types of supplements. Clinical trials now in the final phase of study will make it possible to deliver insulin (a large 140 molecule) orally without injection! This is additional evidence that HGH does pass through the oral areas under the tongue and in the sides of the cheeks.

I prefer to have the biochemical levels of a 20 to 25 year old instead of that of a 44-year-old. I feel like I am humming and people tell me that I look much younger than my years. I would encourage people to recognize that a 35-year-old's levels could be as deficient as that of a 70-year-old. Five percent of the people under 40 years old have deficient IGF levels. Past the age of 65, over half of all men and women who appear to be healthy are dangerously deficient in HGH with IGF levels less than 350 IU. They could decline to as low as under 50 ng/ml. The lowest my IGF levels dropped to was 176 ng/ml that is very low for a person of my age and obviously low compared to youthful levels. Have more than one blood test to take into account the normal variation or fluctuation in hormone levels. It's best to not be too high or too low. Compare your range. The ideal levels would be somewhere between 350 and 450. Both Shawna and I have achieved those levels and continue to maintain them simply by taking the oral HGH replacement.

A great advantage in using **oral HGH** is the convenience of frequent use during the day and evening. To mimic the body, HGH is secreted from the pituitary gland in pulses as often as 9 to 29 times per 24-hour period. Most of the activity and release into the body occurs during the late afternoon and night especially during early hours of sleep. HGH stimulates the production of IGF-1 (as well as other growth factors) which account for most of the anabolic effects of building the body.

Under healthy conditions, the large white cells that migrate in the tissues, called *macrophages*, secrete **growth factors** such as IGF-1, PDGF (platelet-derived growth factor, TGFB1 (Transforming growth factor-beta 1), GM-CSF (granulocyte-macrophage colony stimulating factor) and acidic and basic fibroblast growth factors. These growth factors all regulate cell growth and repair. Cellular repair and the building up of the body's lean mass require protein anabolism and recovery from early inflammatory responses. Healing involves both proper immune system functioning; energy producing processes, and cell to cell communication to avoid muscle wasting associated with age. For example, when lean body mass is reduced to 65% of the ideal body weight, life can no longer be supported and death will occur.

**Benefits of using HGH**

I would like to review with you some other improvements that have been noted in the literature. There have been literally thousands of medical journals that have tracked the results of people using this revolutionary healthy aging treatment with homeopathic HGH and growth factors. Chronic viral infections including herpes simplex, cytomegalovirus, hepatitis viral, coxsackie B, Epstein bar virus, HIV type wasting, leukemia, adenocarcinoma, and diabetes have been helped by competing with viruses for the same genetic sites.

From his breakthrough pioneer work in 1986 using recombinant HGH on a group of elderly patients, and as Dr. Rudman reported in the medical journals; less cellulite, less wrinkles, thicker skin and collagen, sharper vision, and improved memory. The results included increased energy, better exercise performance, cardiac output improvements, a stronger heart, stronger bones to reverse the conditions of osteoporosis, wounds healing more rapidly, an overall 8.8% gain in muscle mass and a body fat reduction of nearly 14.4%, and re-growth of organs. In fact as we get older the liver, the spleen, the kidneys and the heart all decline in size and volume. I have noticed in athletes, especially body builders, when they are taking high levels of injectable HGH, sometimes the abdomen enlarges in size a little bit. That happens because they are actually restoring the size of their organs.

A further great accomplishment of HGH is that it has been shown to lower **LDL cholesterol**, the *bad* cholesterol. You have to take a moment to understand how important a breakthrough this is. LDL is the cholesterol that forms the plaques in the arteries. **Heart attacks** and **strokes** kill more Americans than all other causes combined. So if we have a natural way to help people bring their cholesterol levels down, it can actually help to dissolve the plaques in arteries and restore the arteries to more youthful healthful levels. This is a tremendous breakthrough. I have been working with patients over the last 25 years and have written 6 books, which emphasized how to lower cholesterol with several recipes. I noticed that people as they got older, even with good healthful cholesterol free recipes rich in dietary fiber, many times their cholesterol level went up with age. I couldn't account for this for any other reason because we monitored their food records and we knew they were on a zero cholesterol diet.

Oral HGH replacement is a great way to help restore the youthfulness of the arteries, because it lowers the bad LDL cholesterol. What does that mean? It means that we probably can irradicate and reduce the incidence of heart attacks and strokes with a change in diet, through the natural fibers that do lower cholesterol and by restoration of hormone therapy. We know that lower blood pressure has been accomplished through restoring HGH. Many doctors have reported HGH caused improvements in the elasticity of the arteries and circulation reducing the levels of blood pressure.

Dr. Chin and Dr. L. Cass Terry did some studies on 200 patients during the years of 1994 - 1996. They monitored these people and measured their levels for hormone baseline and they found that these people were low and deficient in HGH as well as some of the other critical hormones. They decided to restore those hormones with the patient's consent. These individuals improved dramatically in the following areas. In fact the improvements measured across the board from 51% to 88% in energy. Improvements in emotional status, in sexual performance, in attitude, in memory, and skin texture improved as well. The skin thickness and elasticity increased, as well as the reported disappearance of wrinkles was also noted. Muscle strength improved, the size of the muscles increased, body fat was reduced, and as well as an increase in exercise tolerance and endurance. All improved using natural hormone replacement therapy. This was recorded in less than a two-year period in individuals past the age of 40.

## Loss of sexual function

We have been hearing a lot in the press about a prescription drug used for sexual performance and we recognize what a critical problem this is in millions of men who have developed sexual impotency. Impotency is a very common problem in our country mainly because of clogged arteries and high cholesterol that narrow the arteries to the male organ. Diabetes, nerve damage or blood pressure medications can cause impotency. The medications reduce blood flow so much that a man can't achieve an erection.

The prescription drug, Viagra is a method to regain short-term sexual potency by providing extra blood flow to the penis. It could cause side effects such as headaches, changes in vision and even risk of death in some frail people. The drug is a temporary solution to an alarm sign that aging is setting in prematurely. Correct the weakness caused by aging and you can restore potency and vitality.

## Sexual Dysfunction and Solutions

Getting to the cause of the problem can solve these physical disorders leading to impotency. Avoidance of foods high in cholesterol like meat, chicken, fish, eggs, and cheese replaced with fresh vegetables, fruit, rice, beans and sprouts in the diet along with HGH replacement and testosterone will unclog arteries to the male organ and restore circulation throughout the body. It would be best to overcome the most common causes of sexual dysfunction by correcting the diet and hormones. Improved blood sugar control will reduce the incidence of diabetes. Over 65% of those on blood pressure medications can be off medicines and back to normal within 30 days using the Healthy Aging plan. As blood flow is restored men can regain sexual potency.

**Hormones restore or improve sexual function in men & women**
Depressed hormone levels is yet another cause of impotency. When the men past the age of 40 in Dr. Chin & Terry's study, restored their hormone levels, the men reported a 75% increase in sexual frequency and potency to achieve erection and a 62% increase in duration of penile erection. Numerous men are reporting similar results within 90 days of using oral HGH and herbs to restore testosterone, enhance libido and desire to have sex. HGH improves performance or the ability to have an erection and sustain it for intercourse. I can tell you that by simply restoring men's hormone levels, phenomenal results can be achieved. Women also improve when given HGH. They reported more interest in sex and enjoyment of sexual orgasms as well as more lubrication offsetting the vaginal dryness associated with aging. 58% of the women reported less hot flashes and 39% improvement in menstrual cycle regulation.

**Aging is a correctable disease**
People who produce little or no HGH because they've had their pituitary gland removed or have Pituitary tumors or disease are deficient in HGH and age rapidly. They have a reduced sense of well being, lower energy, vitality and capacity for work. They exhibit poor memory, mood swings, anxiety, depression and feel socially isolated. Their body fat increases especially around the waist. They have a decrease in muscle mass and wrinkled, thin, prematurely damaged or aged skin. Dr. Bengtsson in Sweden studied 333 patients for 30 years who were diagnosed with pituitary insufficiency. They were given cortisone, thyroid and sex hormones without HGH. The human growth hormone (HGH) deficient patients died prematurely of cardiovascular disease twice as often as the general population. In studies in Denmark and England with patients deficient in HGH after only six months of replacement patients showed improvements both physically and mentally. Once people start the treatment they don't want to stop. Friends and relatives also notice the differences of healthy aging therapy.

**How to stop aging and begin health aging**
Our aging pituitary gland has the ability to release as much HGH compared to when we were younger only if the gland is adequately stimulated. Somatostatin is a substance that increases with age and inhibits or blocks the secretion of HGH. Also as we age, the regulator

GH-RH (Human growth hormone-releasing hormone) that stimulates the release of HGH, becomes less sensitive to our bodies requests or signals for HGH. Another problem is our body tissues and organs become less able to utilize HGH action.

Aging is a disease of the inability to use HGH similar to insulin resistance that occurs with type II diabetes. With Diabetes studies prove that excess fat in the diet desensitizes the insulin receptor sites so insulin can no longer help push sugar into the cells. When you decrease fat in the diet, insulin becomes efficient and able to push sugar into cells as needed, reducing blood sugar levels. Reducing calorie intake increases HGH levels.

**The Healthy aging diet enhances reverses aging**
Years ago, Arnold Schwazenegeer was in a movie called *"Staying Hungry"*. It was about competitive body builders and Arnold pursued his goal of being the best by staying hungry for success, always striving to be the best, never becoming complacent or overly satisfied. Arnold would say "to be muscular and have a low bodyfat you must stay hungry! Don't overeat, eat less calories than you think you need and always be slightly hungry." Obesity suppresses HGH secretion. Research shows that restricting calories will restore the IGF-1 receptors in the cells by as much as 100% as you grow older. Eating small meals only when your hungry and reducing fat can do this. You should eat a water rich diet of vegetables, salads, vegetable soups, and fruit while avoiding meat, oil, dairy products, cheese, eggs and butter. One day a week it would be best to take in blended vegetable and fruit drinks of 32 to 64 oz. in the morning, afternoon and evening. This cleansing can increase HGH levels dramatically. To reverse the disease called aging and slow the signs of age, combine diet and exercise with HGH and HGH releasers to achieve youthful levels.

**Intense exercise** at 70 to 85% of maximum lift during weight lifting and aerobic exercises like running, stair stepping, stationary biking or treadmill at 40 to 70 percent of maximum oxygen uptake, improves the release and efficiency of HGH. I have enjoyed training with weights ever since I was 12 years old. For more than thirty years I have worked out to stay strong, fit and to look better. I work out at least three to five times a week. Aerobics before or after weight training gives me more energy.

Exercise increases the rate at which you can burn fat. Now we have learned that training increases HGH and IGF-1 levels.

## Other ways to stimulate the release of HGH

The history of biochemical hormone replacement included movie stars and athletes traveling to Europe and Mexico to obtain the Fountain of Youth for HGH levels. The use of the vitamin B3 at 250 mg to 1,000 mg a day helps release HGH. A deep sleep REM stages 1, 2, 3 and 4 is less achievable with age. HGH releasers help to restore the deepest stages of sleep. At the deepest levels of sleep we experience rejuvenation and increased levels of HGH. You will begin to wake up totally restored and energized. This is why Melatonin improves sleep because it augments the release of HGH.

## Supplements release HGH & increase IGF

Oral growth Secretagogues are supplements that increase the release of HGH. Amino acids from soy protein isolate like L-Glutamate, L-Arginine L-Ornithine, and Pituitary Complex such as Gamma Aminobutyric Acid with Lacuna Bean Extract(enhances natural L-dopa) release HGH when taken one hour prior to bedtime. The Gamma Aminobutyric Acid (GABA) acts to significantly stimulate the release of HGH. GABA is a neurotransmitter that regulates the pituitary gland to secrete HGH with a 5% increase. This can restore IGF-1 levels a measurement of HGH activity by as much as 10 to 23 percent. The best results were obtained when the amino acids such as L-Lysine and Arginine were combined together at dosages of 1,200 mg to 2,000 mg and taken orally. L-Arginine helps defeat the somatostatin which blocks the release of HGH. The use of L-Arginine is most important in people in their 60's or older when somatostatin increases. Glutamine at 2,000 mg (2 grams) or a ½ teaspoon raised HGH levels four times greater than those given placebo, according to Dr. Welbourne. In people age 32 to 64 the response was equally good at all ages, reported in 1995 the *American Journal of Clinical Nutrition Vol. 61.* Gamma Oryzanol or ferulic acid in double blind studies increased strength, physical performance, lean mass, and reduced cholesterol levels. Dibencozide (coenzyme B-12) helps to synthesize protein and build new muscle tissue while helping one to feel less tired. L-Orinithine Alpha-Ketoglutarate (OKG) has been found to boost gluamine levels more than Glutamine by itself and prevent catabolic breakdown of muscles.

Doctors have reported up to 30% increase in IGF-1 levels using combinations of amino acids such as L-Glutamine, Arginine, GABA, and the vitamin niacin. A 10 to 20% increase in IGF-1 level can have a definite positive effect on the body. Take these combined amino acid with vitamin products on an empty stomach or 4 hours after a meal just before bedtime. It's best to take one day off a week, and one to four weeks off per every three months to prevent the body from adapting. By stopping and starting again you can keep the body responding and maintain your goal of improved IGF-1 levels. You can expect noticeable results of rejuvenation within one to two months and big changes within six months in regards to fat reduction and feeling energized.

**Stress increases cortisol & depresses HGH**

Stress is one of the worst depressors of HGH because of the increase levels of Cortisone. Cortisone is released during times of stress from loss of jobs, divorces, remarriages, deaths in families, or excessive exercise. Small levels of cortisone is necessary to good health, however excess levels will cause catabolic breakdown of muscle tissue, premature aging, and a decline in HGH levels. The cause of stress must first be addressed. Use meditation, attend counseling, avoid negative stressful people, avoid alcohol, and coffee. Allow for additional time for sleep and or naps. Supplement with small dosages of DHEA in conjunction with HGH to counterbalance cortisone and the effects of stress.

**Safe use of natural oral HGH**

Take biochemical hormones sensibly in low dosages. The use of sublingual HGH allows delivery to mimic the bodies natural release into your own system. This is safe because even if you accidentally used the whole bottle of HGH all at one time, you would be ingesting no more than 5,000 ng/ml to 20,000 ng/ml. Now if this sounds like a lot, it actually is not, because Nanograms are a very small measurement of billionths! Furthermore if this amount were ingested at one time it would only be wasted and or excreted, because the body can only use small amounts at daily intervals. It is virtually impossible to cause any side effects with these homeopathic dosages. The obvious safe guard is the product should only be used by those past the age of 25, unless under a doctors guidance, and not for use by pregnant or nursing women.

## Professional & Olympic athletes use HGH

The use of HGH by Olympic Athletes is quite common, because generally speaking there is no current test to detect if an athlete is using HGH injections, or oral supplements.   Anabolic steroids are easily detected by testing and are banned for use by Olympic athletes. Ben Johnson had his record disqualified because of testing positive with steroids. The injection was made into scar tissue and stayed longer in his system then the expected time and he failed his urine test. The female athletes apparently use a bulb of urine from a friend placed in the vagina and squeeze at the time of drug testing. The popular use of HGH by athletes was reported in *Time Magazine* during the last Olympics. New records were set because of the stimulating muscular growth factors of biochemical replacements. Unfortunately, some athletes have abused the use of HGH with injectables. Excessive use of 20 iu's a day can result in hypertrophy of the heart and damage of heart valves.    Stress Echocardiogram can detect early stages of heart problems.  Oral HGH is in safe low dosages of less than 50 ng/ml with further homeopathic dilution. It's used in competition because it is considered by athletes to be a nutritional supplement and safe to use.

## Side effects of high dosage injection of HGH

The only reported side effects were in individuals taking too high of a dosage using injectable HGH. If we compare the high dosage used by injection the use is about one quarter to one I.U. or 250,000 nanograms per I.U.  Bodybuilders and athletes have used as much as 30 to 100 I.U.'s per week while the normal dosage of injectable HGH Nutrophin is between 4 I.U. to 12 I.U.'s per week. Excessive use of HGH can lead to a risk of Acromegaly-or giantism with pronounced forehead, jaw line, and larger nose and feet. Giantism would take over 30 years to develop using excessive dosages of injectable.   Carpal tunnel syndrome-painful stiff joints from excess fluid retention can occur in people not exercising. Reduced  dosage  and  more  frequent  use  reversed  the  problem. Gynecomastia (enlarged breasts in men) is much less common. High dose, long term use of HGH can cause insulin resistance, diabetes, arthritis and hypertension. If side effects appeared the individuals were asked to reduce the dosage until the side effects disappeared.

By using the natural oral HGH or stimulators of human growth factors, as IGF-1 increases and tissue rehydration occurs, some people report slight ache in the wrist or shoulder. This will pass soon, especially if you are exercising to prevent fluid retention and following a low-fat, low-salt diet. This added water in the organs and muscles of the body would improve your strength and performance doing your daily activities.

**Less cancer in acromegaly caused by HGH**

According the *Journal of Clinical Endocrinology & Metabolism*, August 1998, Volume 83, In acromegaly with excessive levels of HGH in their system present during most of their life. "The overall cancer incidence rate (new cancers at any site in the body including breast, thyroid, colon, lung, or prostate) was lower than that in the general population in the United Kingdom. The overall mortality death rate was not increased when compared to the general population. Death rate from colon cancer and cardiovascular heart disease was slightly higher than the expected rate for the general population. If HGH were a risk for cancer, you would expect a higher rate of new cancers at all sites and a higher death rate from all types of cancer. The findings reported less cancers in people with high HGH levels than those compared to people with normal HGH levels! From this information, HGH and IGF1 replaced at ideal levels would not increase the risk of cancer; it may add a protective factor.

**HGH build immune-system-fight cancer?**

Is it possible that HGH and IGF-1 may reduce the risk of cancer? Cancer becomes more dangerous as a risk with age. Cancer is considered the second leading cause of death in the United States following heart disease, stroke and heart attack. One of the important factors to overcome or reduce the incidence of cancer is our own bodies' immune system. We have the ability to reduce the risk of cancer by maintaining the blood in a slightly alkaline state with diet and supplements and by enhancing our own immune factors and lymphatic system. The lymphatic system has a very extensive circulating system throughout the body. If you were to take the whole lymphatic system together it is a greater system and takes up more mass and more fluid volume than the entire blood stream in your body. How efficient are your lymphatic system, your white cells and your killer T cells?

What if you have depressed IGF-1 and HGH levels? We know the answer to this because with age, there is a decline in hormone levels as compared to when you were younger and an increase in the incidence of cancer. How could this be? Clearly as we restore or increase the levels of HGH we would expect a decline in the risk of cancer. It is true that IGF-1 increases above normal levels in people with deficient levels, after someone develops cancer. This increase in IGF-1 is to cope with the inflammation caused from cancerous tumors. The increased IGF-1 could not possibly have caused the cancer, otherwise you would see a high incidence of cancer in young children and yet we see the opposite. The decreased risk of cancer is associated with a strong immune system and higher youthful levels of HGH, as well as DHEA, Melatonin, and testosterone. A lot of exciting research is now under way with these various hormones to fight cancer.

As I looked further through the literature there were reports of restoring Melatonin levels to help fight cancer. Dr. Edmund Chin and L. Cass Terry's researched over 800 people ranging in age from 40 to 74, who had their HGH levels restored to youthful levels. You would have thought that we would have seen some incidence of cancer just because of their advanced age, however we discovered absolutely no evidence of cancer in all 800 people.

One patient who had a proven case of prostate cancer was warned that there was no way of knowing what would happen with hormone therapy. The patient requested the youth restoring hormone therapy to see if it might help his condition. When they restored the IGF-1 levels the prostate cancer improved according to the PSA levels and follow up biopsies. Blood testing on other patients given hormone therapy showed the PSA levels were reduced and had less risk of prostate cancer. According to this preliminary evidence, I would predict we will find an overall decline in cancer rates when we examine middle-aged and senior citizens who have restored these hormone levels to youthful levels.

I hope you are convinced to have your hormone levels checked for IGF-1 and human growth hormone (HGH, somatomedin C). You want to feel and experience what everyone is talking about regarding HGH and IGF-1, don't you? Have your levels rechecked within eight weeks of using the oral HGH and IGF-1 replacements. Be consistent about your exercise and diet. You will feel the excitement of being proactive about your life and experience what healthy aging is all about.

# II

∞

# Fountain of Youth

---

Anti-aging, preserving our youth and reverse aging is a hot topic because it affects all of us. The people most interested in looking and feeling younger represent a growing segment of "Baby Boomers" past the age of 35. Visit a retirement home or convalescent hospital and you will see the ravages of aging in our senior citizens. By the year 2030 we will have 52 million Americans past the age of 70.

Some people age more rapidly than others, because of a breakdown in our body's aging clock. Our organs age, shrink in size and produce fewer hormones. This reduction in available hormones leads to a slow deterioration of all of our vital body systems. The declines in the Immune system, Reproductive, Neurological, Metabolic and Circulatory systems cause us to look and feel old.

The "Fountain of Youth" involves understanding the aging process. There are eight critical hormones that decrease, as we grow older causing us to age rapidly. Reversing the clock is a matter of simply restoring these eight hormones to your youthful levels. I have seen numerous examples of people looking and feeling ten to twenty years younger within only ninety days. Total replacement of all the deficient hormones is new, however hormone replacement therapy has been around for years. All of the hormones replaced have been in our bodies and have been replenished by endocrinologists for decades. Finally we are realizing the necessity to replace all of the hormones at the same time to a more optimal physiologic level.

**Any deficient hormones require natural supplementation**
The results I obtained with HGH led me on to the pursuit of analyzing each of the critical hormones. I had my levels measured for DHEA, Human growth factors by IGF-1 and HGH, *Total* Testosterone & *Free*

Testosterone, melatonin, pregenolone, thyroid, progesterone and estrogen. Each of these levels should be checked very carefully because with aging, there are certain optimum levels that we need to maintain.

**Pregnenolone** also known as Preg is considered the Grandmother hormone because it can be converted by the body into DHEA and Progesterone and over 150 other important natural steroid hormones. Preg helps keep our brains functioning at peak capacity. It is a potent memory enhancer that improves concentration, fights mental fatigue, depression and reduces arthritis. According to Ray Sahelian M.D., many people reported that Pregnenolone provided as much alertness as coffee. It made them more focused yet relaxed. Pregnenolone must be taken in the morning because it increases alertness, mental clarity and heightened awareness. It is best not to take at night because it could cause insomnia. It will enhance and possibly increase levels of DHEA and progestrone. Pregnenolone is produced from cholesterol. DHEA, testosterone, and estrogen are also made from cholesterol. Low cholesterol levels will not interfere with the maintenance of proper normal levels. However, as we age the ability to convert cholesterol to proper hormonal levels is a problem. Take supplements providing 2-10 mg per day to replace what you need to restore your levels. For people past the age of 50 you may take up to 15 mg per day. Be sure to stay on low dosages of Pregnenolone. At dosages over 25 mg per day some people complain of irritability, headaches or insomnia. At low dosages you may expect enhanced mood, euphoria, alertness and energy. Pregnenolone adult blood levels should range between 20-150 ng/100ml or for Preg Sulfate 2.7-8 mcg/100 ml. Preg concentrates in the brain and central neural tissues over 70 times more that in the blood. DHEA is only 6 times higher in the brain than blood, with more found in the peripheral tissues.

**DHEA** is a critical hormone, which controls several other important hormones, including serotonin, testosterone, progesterone, and estrogen. The need for this hormone, DHEA Dehydroepiandrosterone (De-hydro-epi-an-DROS-ter-own) is undeniable. DHEA is a hormone that can be transformed into almost any other hormone, as the body needs it. DHEA is concentrated in the brain six times more than in any other tissue or organ. Humans produce the largest amount of DHEA as compared to other primates or other animals. Every tissue of the human body has enzymes necessary for the metabolism of DHEA. DHEA is produced in the adrenals, ovaries, testicles and brain.

At this time, studies by Dr. Yen suggest that we may replace some of the drop in HGH with DHEA. There was a 10% increase in Insulin like Growth Factor (IGF-1) levels and a 19% decline in Binding Protein (IGFBP-1) creating a 50% ratio improvement. This was the benefit of taking 50 mg of DHEA nightly for six months.

Dr. Cranton MD has been carefully monitoring patients on small amounts of DHEA for over five years. He gave the example of a forty one-year-old man who had low levels for his age. After a few months on DHEA, his blood levels of DHEA were restored to youthful levels. He noticed his energy level was markedly higher. His skin was thicker and moister, and he was sleeping six and half-hours a night instead of eight and waking rested. He felt six or seven years younger, his sex drive increased significantly, and he said, "When you're on DHEA, it feels as if every cell in your body is just humming."

A female patient with Asthma experienced astonishing results, she said, "Within an hour after taking my first capsule of DHEA ' I suddenly found I could breathe again. That month my periods, which had been irregular, went back to normal-I was on my old regular twenty-seven day cycle-and my headaches disappeared. My depression lifted within the first few days. Two months after I started DHEA I joined a dance class. It had always been a childhood dream to dance. I feel like a teenager, as if I were renewing myself."

Dr. Yen reported in *the Journal of Clinical Endocrinology and Metabolism 1994* giving men and women age 40 to 70 years old, DHEA (50 mg taken orally) at bedtime for 6 months. In two weeks the blood levels of DHEA were restored to youthful levels (double blind, placebo crossover study). There was a remarkable increase in perceived physical and psychological well being in 67% of the men and 84% of the women. The participants said they slept better, had more energy, and handled stress better, with no side effects. DHEA helps maintain the immune system, providing a protein sparing effect while improving levels.

Benefits of DHEA, according to over 2,500 published papers, are DHEA decreases abnormal platelet aggregation and LDL ("bad")

41

cholesterol levels. This reduces the risk of heart attacks and stroke. DHEA enhances the immune system and the thymus gland, reduces the rate of infection, Epstein Bar, Lupus, herpes and cancer. DHEA reduces the stress hormone cortisol and helps offset caffeine and the catabolic effects of exercise. DHEA increases serotonin naturally, which decreases food consumption and helps speed weight loss, according to *The Journal of Clinical Endocrinology and Metabolism 1995.*

People taking higher amounts of DHEA (1,500 mg per day) for 28 days have reduced body fat by as much as 31% with an equal gain in muscle mass, and no loss of weight. DHEA helps to burn excess calories instead of storing glycogen. Obese people tend to have higher insulin levels. DHEA helps to lower insulin levels by pushing glucose into your cells to be burned. DHEA helps reduce appetite by creating a feeling of "fullness".

DHEA is available as capsules, tablets, liquid sublingual under the tongue or transdermal cream applied to the skin. Precursors of DHEA from wild yam do not convert very well into DHEA, so I prefer to use the actual DHEA pharmaceutical grade. I don't believe you should take such high dosages of this powerful hormone. It would be better to take DHEA in very small dosages of less than 25 mg a day, or in liposomal cream or spray form require less than 2 mg a day. You only need 2 mg in cream or spray because of superior absorption. Stay with these low dosages and allow your body time to adjust and build up gradually to avoid possible side effects of excess use of DHEA. Dr. Bill Timmins suggests you also monitor day and evening Cortisol levels.

DHEA has many of the **benefits of estrogen**, with little or no side effects. It helps women with vaginal atrophy to stimulate the cellular growth of the vaginal wall, increased vaginal secretion, thus restoring the vagina to its youthful condition. Studies on female cancer patients that had ovaries removed reported little or no change in sex drive. The ovaries produce estrogen and testosterone. However, after removal of the Adrenal glands, the site of DHEA production, four out of five women experienced a total loss of sexual desire and responsiveness. A combination of DHEA and Free Testosterone are the most important hormones for sexual interest and desire in women.

DHEA produces the **pheromones** that emit our scent through the skin. Pheromones act on our brain to receive the scent of the *opposite sex*. It may influence our choice of mate, if we become pregnant, and the bonding with our babies. DHEA is produced by the fetus two hundred to eight hundred times higher than the levels of progesterone, testosterone, and estrogen.

This tremendous amount of DHEA present during youth has intrigued longevity researchers. DHEA drops to near zero in all people at death. Will we **prolong life** an additional ten or twenty years if we take supplements of DHEA to maintain youthful levels? Studies show that an increase in blood levels of DHEA sulfate is associated with a 36% less mortality rate from any cause.

DHEA **declines** from heavy alcohol drinking, birth control pills, stress, hypothyroidism, and lack of exercise and obesity. More is not necessarily better in the case of hormone replacement. **High dosages** of DHEA (1,600 mg a day) can cause acne, unwanted hair growth, irritability, headaches, and rapid heart beat. If you are having any side effects, reduce the dosage gradually down to lower intakes. Have your DHEA levels checked by saliva tests to monitor your progress and maintain ideal levels.

Stay within the safe guidelines for anti-aging of 25 mg capsule or 2 mg spray a night for women and 25 mg (2 mg spray) morning & night for men. Some people take up to 100 mg of DHEA a day to reach ideal levels, however, these higher dosages should be monitored monthly by both saliva and blood with your health professional. The goal is to bring **DHEA sulfate** and **Free DHEA** combined, to youthful levels of a person aged 20 to 25. **Saliva DHEA for men** is best at 10.9 to 16.9 Nmol/L or 200 to 300 pg./ml. Ideal for **women** is 7.2 to 8.5 Nome/L or 125 to 170 pg./ml. **Blood tests** for serum DHEA goal is 300 to 400 mg/dl for **women** and 450 to 600 mg/dl for **men**. Ideal levels for DHEA (Free unbound) is 700 to 1200 ng/dl for men and 450 to 800 ng/dl for women.

③ The next critical hormone that slows aging is **testosterone**. Free & total testosterone is found naturally circulating in the bloodstream of baby boys creating the male testes and penis. Small amounts of testosterone produced in women's ovaries and adrenals provide energy, libido and a feeling of well being. Young teenagers and adult men have large increases in free testosterone followed by a gradual decrease after age 30. Free testosterone becomes bound and unusable as we age by Sex Hormone Binding Globulin (SBBG).

A 73-year-old Doctor said, "I take testosterone because I want to feel the same way I did when I was in my prime. I want to have the same sexuality that I did when I was young. I want to maintain my muscle strength. I want to feel vital. Testosterone makes it all possible."

Research during W.W II on testosterone showed the powerful effect on the immune system. A physician transplanted testes from a dying soldier into the abdomen of a soldier suffering from gangrene caused by a gunshot wound. The soldier would have died, but the gangrene was cured following the transplant of the testes. In 1934 a scientist isolated the testosterone make up and received the Nobel Prize. Discoveries in 1951 reported that testosterone improves nitrogen balance, increases muscle mass and repairs damaged bones and ligaments.

In the 1960's it was discovered that testosterone lowers cholesterol, improves abnormal EKG's of cardiac patients, helps claudication (clogged leg arteries) and angina pectoris (chest pain) -clogged heart arteries. Free testosterone maintained at youthful levels protects men against atherosclerosis -hardening of the arteries. Testosterone also improves diabetic retinopathy, helping eyesight, lowers insulin requirements and enhances glucose tolerance of diabetic patients.

Testosterone decreases body fat, improves waist-to-hip ratio of fat and enhances lean body mass. It has a protective effect against autoimmune diseases such as lupus and rheumatoid arthritis. Studies show that men with high testosterone levels live longer, healthier lives and maintain sexual potency. Men over 50 years old with low testosterone levels, in a double blind, placebo-controlled study, were given either replacement testosterone for 90 days or a placebo. They found the hormone renewed strength, improved balance and increased libido. Restoring testosterone increased red blood cell count, lowered LDL ("bad") cholesterol and enhanced feelings of well being.

In *July 1996 New England Journal of Medicine* researchers discovered that testosterone significantly enhanced muscle size and reduced body fat even in men who do not exercise or go on a diet. Three groups of male weight lifters did the same exercise or no exercise. The men were given testosterone or placebo every week for ten weeks. The men given testosterone had much more muscle whether or not they exercised.

The *American Journal of Physiology* reported in men age 67 after only 4 weeks with the addition of testosterone an increase in leg muscle strength and restored muscle size. In another study at the University of Washington, men past the age of 60 who were given testosterone for three months lost fat and gained muscle without going on a diet!

Crossover studies where the placebo group was given testosterone, and the group given testosterone was taken off, men reported being more aggressive and energetic at work. The men with normalized testosterone levels found that their relationships improved with their wives because of better sexual performance, initiation of sexual intercourse and increased ability to maintain an erection.

In older men, ages 31 to 80, high levels of Sex Hormone Binding Globulin reduced free testosterone in 74% of the men complaining of sexual dysfunction. Nearly 80% of the men had a reduction in **libido** (interest in sex), difficulty in getting or maintaining an **erection**, rarely had early **morning erections** and 92% experienced a reduction in **sexual satisfaction**.

In addition, these men with low free testosterone levels reported fatigue, depression, irritability, aches, pains and stiffness. A significant drop in free testosterone can occur as early as age 40. At age 60, 18% of men are impotent and at age 80, 75% are impotent. Once a man becomes impotent he loses his drive for life, has impaired erections, his muscles become thinner, he becomes depressed and mental acuity fade.

All healthy males get **erections**, mostly during the REM dream stage of sleep every night without exception. These erections are not stimulated or associated with the content of dreams. The penis of a medically fit man erects more than 10 times a night! Erections occur in cycles lasting about 30 minutes, although the penis is not fully erect the entire time.

If a man wakes up in the middle of the night with an erection this is a normal healthy sign. If he gets an erection early in the morning, he can rest assured that his penis is in good working order. If he is not having good erections during sex, any difficulty is probably psychological. That is assuming random erections occur. You can do a simple test using postage stamps to test for erections. Take a roll of postage stamps and wrap it around the flaccid penis before sleep. If the perforations between the stamps tear by morning, then the man had an erection during the night. If no erection, then the problem is organic and physical.

The following 3 tests can determine what type organic problem exists:

1. **Vascular disorders** are the most common causes of penile erection dysfunction. High cholesterol levels will clog arteries that bring blood to the penis or by leaks in the venous system that result when the blood in the shaft of the penis drains out prematurely. A doctor can use one simple injection of vasoactive drugs (Papaverine or Prostaglandin-E) to determine whether the arterial system is intact. The drug produces an immediate erection in healthy men regardless of the mental factor. The penis either gets hard or it does not. If it does not, then you need to clean the arteries. Change to a cholesterol free vegetarian diet, take soluble fibers, reduce alcohol, stop smoking, especially before sex, increase free testosterone to reduce atherosclerosis and see a doctor for treatment.

2. The test for **neurological problems** is performed by inserting a gloved finger one-inch into the man's anus to feel the sphincter muscle and with the other hand gently squeezing the tip of the penis. If the nerves to the penis are working properly, squeezing the tip of the penis will cause the anal sphincter to contract firmly against the finger.

3. **Hormonal disorders** are the third common cause of erection failure. Diabetes, overactive or under-active thyroid and low HGH levels can cause erection failure. Lack of testosterone can also cause erection failure. Saliva or blood can test these hormone disorders. Restoring hormone levels to normal levels can solve these erection problems.

The **herbs** Avena Sativa (Green Oats), Nettles, and Saw Palmetto can restore free testosterone to the youthful range for men and women. One

46

gram per day of the B-Vitamin niacin also reportedly helps lower Sex Hormone Binding Globulin and releases the free testosterone. Another supplement, Testron SX, and the mineral zinc, has been reported to increase natural testosterone production. Testron SX also helps keep DHT (dihydrotestosterone) in a free state, non binding. In most people, the natural herbs and vitamins restore youthful levels. In some people, replacement therapy with gel or transdermal testosterone may be necessary. This can improve the quality of life for adults.

To enhance testosterone **Tribulus terrestris fruit** extract at 1,000 to 2,000 mg dosage helps LH factor to increase testosterone. Avena Sativa, which is, sprouted green oats, and the herb nettles removes sex hormone binding globulin and releases free testosterone. Saw Palmetto prevents the conversion of testosterone to deyhdrotestosterone. This helps to avoid the any negative affects of acne, balding or masculinzing effects. Zinc increases total testosterone production.

**Androstenedione** supplements gained national attention when it was reported that "home run king" Mark McGwire hit a record 70 home runs in a single season for 1998, while taking this amazing supplement to increase testosterone. Androstenedione can boost strength, muscular size, and endurance. Oral use of 50 to 100 mg.-raised testosterone levels over 200%. This was over twice as effective as DHEA in raising testosterone. Androstenedione should only be taking before athletic events, or before sex and not more than three times a week. If overused, the excess production of testosterone can convert into too much estrogen and reverse your benefits.

**Salivary** testosterone levels ideal for men are 200 to 400 pmol/L. Men with saliva levels less than 120 pmol/L can benefit from supplements. Free testosterone blood levels for men should be 19 to 40 pg./ml. Men with low levels of 1 to 9 pg./ml could benefit from supplement therapy. Ideal **blood** levels for total testosterone for men is 500 to 1200 Ng/dl (nanograms per deciliter). Men with low levels of less than 400 Ng/dl bearing watching and under 250 Ng/dl need treatment. If you restore these low testosterone levels to what they should be you may feel like you were 25 years old again! By the age of 30 free testosterone levels start to drop gradually with age. Have your level checked with a simple saliva test.

Ideal range for women salivary testosterone is 80 to 155 pmol/L. **Blood** tests for free testosterone during ovulation, age 20 to 29 is .9 to 3.9 ng/ml, and total testosterone levels of 16 to 100 Ng/dl. This is the time when women are most fertile. Past the age of 50, postmenopausal women have their lowest blood levels of *free* **testosterone** at .3 to 2.7 pg./ml. Past the age of 40, menopausal women's *total* **testosterone** levels can drop to zero to 64 Ng/dl.

It is best to stay in the youthful range, not too low or too high. Excessive levels of testosterone in women can occur from ovarian or adrenal disorders or excessive dosages of supplements leading to acne, increased body hair growth, deepening of the voice or balding.

The combination of *bound* and *free testosterone* is **total testosterone**. Doctors mistakenly usually only check total testosterone. However, it is the free testosterone that is the only biologically active part from a health and sexual point of view. Even if an adult has total testosterone levels above normal, but has below-normal free testosterone, your sex drive will probably be sluggish and nonexistent. Think of free testosterone as the only active part with high impact on your health. Testosterone significantly increases following resistance exercise workouts. The resting testosterone (hours after exercise) was found to decrease when excess protein was added in the diet. As protein increased, resting testosterone levels decreased. Low fat intake under 10%, decreased testosterone. It is important to use weight training and the recommended herbs and supplements in place of added fat to maintain proper levels of testosterone as you age.

**Saliva tests** for free testosterone and DHEA can be provided by contacting us by sending a stamped return envelope for information to Healthy Studios 25422 Trabuco Road, #105-141 Lake Forest, CA 92630, or call 800-631-0232. We can refer you to those who can provide you a *test kit* that you send back with a fee to have your level of free testosterone and DHEA checked. Saliva tests are easy to collect and mail to the laboratory without involving clinic staff, no biohazard, no mess, and no blood, very convenient and economical.

Saliva tests are accurate with over a 90% correlation to blood tests results. Saliva tests can measure the effects of supplements better than blood, because spinning blood separates out cells that may have 75% of the hormones. Your supplements for testosterone or DHEA may be working, but blood tests may not pick up the improvements as well as Saliva tests. Saliva tests pick up the full tissue levels for hormones. We can measure other important hormones in saliva including melatonin, estradiol, progesterone and cortisol.

Testosterone, estrogen, progesterone and melatonin are cyclic, going up and down throughout the day, night and month. Saliva tests for free testosterone is performed with three samples taken morning, afternoon and late night. A man's testosterone level is highest in the morning. The levels change every 15 minutes. Testosterone can vary by 100 ng (serum) or more with variations from day to day by as much as 50%. By taking a series of samples we can accurately track the average range and a doctor can determine if you need replacement therapy.

My free testosterone increased dramatically within four weeks using herbs ( Avena Sativa, Saw Palmetto, nettles and ionic minerals with zinc) from under 1.3 ng/dl (severely deficient) to over 22 to 28 ng/dl (ideal for a young 20 year old man, yet I'm age 43) based on blood tests.    I experienced a healthy increase in libido, strength and muscle density while taking the herbs.

In another trial, I wanted to test DHEA in spray form.    My free testosterone measured by saliva increase from 49 pg. to 100 pg. after taking 2 mg DHEA three times a day for six days. This was too high, so I learned I could reduce my dosage of DHEA down to one time a day in spray form.    The doctor working with the lab called me about the results because he was amazed by the significant increase.

DHEA sulfate is very stable with very little change in levels from day to day. A single saliva test for DHEA can tell us if your levels are below ideal. We need to take supplements of DHEA to prevent the decline associated with aging. The addition of DHEA can convert into the necessary testosterone, as the body needs. The DHEA and herbs like Avena Sativa may completely restore the free and total testosterone to normal levels in most of the cases. However, if it doesn't normalize your testosterone levels then see your doctor for a prescription of natural, micronized testosterone gel to solve the problem.

Surprisingly it takes very small amounts of testosterone to physically maintain an erection and enjoy sex. The problem is that a man low in testosterone may simply not care enough to pursue it. Once testosterone levels are replenished a man will find that he has recaptured a healthy interest in sex. Men have gone from zero libidos to a vigorous sex life within ten days.

The saying, "if you don't use it you lose it" applies with testosterone. Frequency of sex increases testosterone in both male and females after sex. Salivary testosterone concentrations were measured in a study of four couples on a total of eleven evenings before and after sexual intercourse and eleven evenings when there was no intercourse. Testosterone increased in men and women when there was intercourse and decreased when there was none. Your relationship plays a meaningful role in immunity, health and longevity. This may account way married men, with active sex lives, had higher testosterone levels and live longer than single men.

Women during menopause who have tried hormone replacement with estrogen and progesterone are starting to be given a small amount of testosterone which replenishes energy, libido and feeling good again. Remember, women need testosterone to be healthy and maintain strong bones and proper balance.

Testosterone, HGH, progesterone and DHEA are the ultimate aphrodisiacs. Testosterone along with DHEA is responsible for the sex drive of both men and women; stimulating our desire for sexual activity and orgasm. It is **testosterone**, not estrogen that causes the heightened erotic sensitivity of the clitoris, breasts, and nipples. Testosterone encourages a woman to go after a man. She becomes more sexual, more responsive and more assertive. It does not influence the frequency of intercourse. Testosterone improves self-confidence and serves as an antidepressant in women. Testosterone is regulated by **LHRH-** (Luteinizing Hormone Releasing Hormone), the director of testosterone to give you desires.

**PEA-** (phenylethylamine) is the hormone that releases when you see someone you're interested in causing attraction to the opposite sex. **DHEA**

contributes to the sex drive in both men and women, increasing your libido by sensitizing your erogenous zones to touch and promoting positive sexual scents called **pheromones. Dopamine** increases our receptivity to pleasure. High **serotonin** levels reduce our interest in sex and inhibit orgasm in both sexes. Low serotonin levels caused by diet pills can increase aggression and excessive sexual aberrations.

**Estrogen** is a warm, receptive, willing, passive and seductive hormone. **Progesterone** and **prolactin** are nurturer hormones, reducing sex drive. **Oxytocin** increases during touch creating bonding and a feeling of love. **Vasopressin** is a peptide like hormone that bonds and enhances parenting feelings, according to Dr. Theresa Crenshaw.

By the age of 35, most women have 50% less of this critical hormone **progesterone.** It continues to decrease with age until you are totally deficient. The supplement of natural progesterone in the cream (Eden's Secret from wild yam), has been manufactured to be identical to the female molecule. It is a better choice in place of synthetic progesterone like Progestins or Provera. Many women feel remarkably better using the natural cream or transdermal form of natural progesterone. Natural progesterone and testosterone increases bone density preventing osteoporosis. Estrogen can only slow bone loses.

## REDUCE MENOPAUSE AND PMS SYMPTOMS

Women are using powerful synthetic hormone replacement therapy pills prescribed by doctors and P.M.S. clinics with little regard to the potential long-term serious side effects. These synthetic hormone pills increase the risk of cancer and blood clotting and under prescription. Fortunately, there is an alternative, safe course to follow using diet and exercise. Natural Progesterone with testosterone gel prevents osteoporosis, not estrogen. Evidence showing the slowing of bone loss has been documented. Pharmaceutical UPS grade natural Progesterone cream is non-prescription because it's safe and proven to prevent bone loss and strengthen the bone.

High protein diet, lack of sufficient exercise, and deficient hormones cause osteoporosis. If you start a daily walking program today, with weight training two times a week, you can immediately replace lost bone material. The high complex carbohydrate diet centers meals on vegetables, rice and fruit, instead of around proteins like meat, fish, chicken, milk and cheese. As you follow

51

this lower protein diet your bones will begin to reabsorb lost bone material. You will receive adequate protein from the carbohydrate foods.

Before and after x-rays of people with osteoporosis has demonstrated a strengthening of bones by reducing dietary protein and exercising daily. Urine tests measuring calcium retention have shown immediate improvements of positive calcium balance (more calcium has been absorbed than lost). People on a high protein diet who do not exercise lose more calcium out of the urine than they take in from their diet. Hormone pills by themselves are not the answer - diet and exercise are the key to building bones with age.

**Progesterone cream** rubbed on your skin is absorbed 40 to 70 times more efficiently as compared to a pill. You need only a small quantity of *cream* rubbed into your fatty areas providing 10 mg to 20 mg. To equal this amount, you would have to take 200 to 400 mg as an ***oral pill***, because the pill goes to the liver and is broken down into artificial metabolites. If you take a pill for progesterone (progesterone is fat-soluble) most of it is wasted, because the serum in the blood is water-soluble. You only get from the pill 5% of the 200 mg or 10mg. The progesterone in the cream is absorbed from the skin, directly into the red blood cells and then it reaches the tissues of the body. Red Blood cells have a fatty membrane that allows transport of the progesterone where the body needs it.

A **saliva test** is the best way to measure **progesterone levels**. Saliva is fat-soluble and can transport in the fatty membranes of saliva tissue. Blood serum is water-soluble and it will not show the increased levels from cream. Some doctors were led to believe the creams were less effective than pills based on blood tests. French doctors in 1997 measured breast tissue for progesterone levels and found it increased over 100 times using cream for progesterone. This proved excellent absorption using cream, even though blood levels showed no increase. This is because the transport of progesterone occurred by way of the Red Cells, not the watery blood serum plasma (clear golden fluid). Only 1 to 9 percent of the progesterone bound in proteins is usable coming from pills via the ovaries. Doctors had made the wrong conclusion about cream delivery. They don't even know to check the progesterone level with saliva. Saliva carries the biologically active form of progesterone, DHEA, testosterone, melatonin and estrogen.

For years we have been aware that women have the need for replacement of estrogen and progesterone. Unfortunately, hormone replacement got a bad reputation because of side effects caused by using *synthetic* hormones like Provera, and Premarin to replace estrogen. S*ynthetic* estrogen known as Premarin can cause irritability, fluid retention, and breast tenderness. Pharmaceutical companies developed and patent a replacement using molecules that were not identical to the female estrogen molecules. They could not patent natural triple or bi estrogen, so they produced and marketed synthetic altered molecules called *"conjugated estrogens"* from horse urine! Nearly half of all women using synthetic estrogen stopped because of the concern of side effects reported in many women.

Fat in the diet will cause hormonal imbalances because an overproduction of estrogen. These drastic hormonal imbalances can be corrected by following our low-fat diet, losing weight and by daily, long distance walking exercises. *Synthetic* estrogen hormones tend to cause weight gain by increasing fat production and increasing fluid retention. The Healthy Aging Diet will help by reducing fluid retention and reducing body fat from the hips, thighs and stomach. You will look and feel great each additional month that you closely adhere to the plan.

By using natural plant based estrogen with progesterone supplements, and vaginal cream you can avoid the usual side affects of synthetic hormones. Dr. John Lee says "Never take estrogen of any kind unopposed to progesterone." Always include the use of natural progesterone, DHEA and testosterone to avoid any cancer risk or side effects. The Healthy Aging low-fat diet and exercise plan will also decrease and prevent fibroid tumors, uterine cysts, endometrial thickening and "heavy" periods. Typically the amount of progesterone cream can be reduced and periods are lighter, with little or no bleeding after menopause. Natural Progesterone will play a big role in restoring the imbalance caused by unopposed estrogen according to Dr. John Lee.

You gain all the benefits using natural **Triple estrogen or Bi estrogen** such as **Estriol** at 80 to 90% ratio to **Estradiol** and with or without **Estrone** at 3 to 10%, according to Dr. Jonathan Wright MD. You can expect reduced hot flashes, night sweats, better memory, alertness, and reduced aging of the skin. Natural hormones may also reduce the incidence of Alzheimer's disease, heart disease, and colon cancer. Doctors are now starting to realize that it is really much better to prescribe *natural* **triple estrogen**, to mimic the bodies needs. There are creams and herbs that support estrogen requirements, which you can obtain directly from distributors. The best creams are EsGen and herbs include: PhytoGen-genistein a soy plant estrogen in capsules, herbs that help balance the female hormone are Black Cohosh, Cayenne, Dong Quai, Hawaiian noni, Una De Gato.

We have several women come to one of our referral medical clinics that have stopped taking those synthetic hormone pills and switched to natural hormones and faithfully followed the Healthy aging Diet and Exercise Plan. These women report less fatigue, increased energy and control of mood swings. Many women have been able to avoid hysterectomy surgery as the pain caused by fibroid tumors and uterine cysts disappeared.

**Estrogen** is considered a new weapon against **Alzheimer's,** according the journal *Science, May 2, 1997, Vol. 276.* An 80-year-old woman named Elsa was treated with estrogen by her doctor, Howard Fillit. Prior to treatment, Elsa was quiet, apathetic, and unable to learn pairs of words, even after seeing them dozens of times. Afterward, she was much more alert, talkative, and able to remember the words after just a few times. The treatment with estrogen was so successful Elsa won back her mind and a marriage proposal from her boyfriend. True love was rekindled between her and her boyfriend, a poet. Besides Elsa, two of the six other women in the study also showed gains in their cognitive skills. Sanjay Asthana, and his colleagues in Tacoma, Washington, reported five of six women who had mild Alzheimer's disease and wore an estrogen patch (It would be better to use the safer, natural triple estrogen) for two month showed improvements in verbal memory and attention. "We found a direct relationship between the level of estrogen in the blood and improvement in memory." The effect disappeared when the treated women went off estrogen. The estrogen hormone may cooperate with neurotrophins, potent stimulators of nerve-cell growth in the brain, such as nerve growth factor (NGF).

More and more doctors are starting to ignore advertisements to use synthetic hormones by pharmaceutical companies and they are allowing their patients the safer alternative of hormones derived from plants, wild yams or soy products.

Women are told to use Synthetic hormones for mood changes of depression and irritability just before the menstrual cycles (Premenstrual syndrome) and after menopause. Have your doctor switch you over to natural triple estrogen or bi estrogen, preg and progesterone . This will closely match your body's normal needs.

## Skin younger, less wrinkles

Menopausal women must use natural progesterone cream, preg, DHEA, and plant based triple estrogen creams (from a compound pharmacist), HGH and testosterone to keep the skin "beautiful and young". The following steps are essential and effective for best results:

1. Avoid smoking. Smokers skin wrinkles 10 years sooner than non-smokers do. Carbon monoxide deprives the skin in the face (near the smoke) of oxygen. Look at a smoker and non-smokers face and you'll notice how many more wrinkles the smoker has.

2. Limit exposure to the sun and use the appropriate sunscreens. The excess sun exposure ages and wrinkles the skin. A suntan gives your body a healthy look, but sun bathe only in the early morning or late afternoon for less than 1 hour to avoid overdosing from the sun.

3. DO NOT wash your skin on your face with soap. Any kind of soap dries the skin because it contains sodium hydroxide. Sodium hydroxide is alkaline, which is also used in Drano toilet cleaners and used to remove grease. If you follow a low-fat diet you will not have oily skin. Therefore, you will not need soap on your face. You ask then, what should you use? A former Miss America used fresh, bottled water to rinse her face and body. Keep a bottle near the sink and in the shower. Use the bottled water as a final rinse. Your skin sloughs off old skin every three days. This is your body's' way of cleansing itself. It would be acceptable to use soap under the arms, in the pelvic region and the hands to reduce bacteria and dirt exposure. Use a gentle shampoo, pH balanced, with conditioner on the hair to avoid dry scalp.

Use lotions on your skin to prevent dryness. Your skin will radiate with health as you follow the Healthy Aging low-fat diet. As your blood carries more oxygen, your skin will take on a youthful appearance in addition to adding natural hormones.

There are successful, natural ways to adjust for the decrease of hormone production after menopause. Using vegetable or fruit oils such as coconut, apricot kernel, safflower, baby oil or Vitamin E oil can solve the thinning of vaginal wall tissue. DON'T EAT THE OIL -Have your spouse apply it to the length of your vagina. K-Y Jelly can be used, but it may dry too quickly. Avoid oils containing alcohol, Vaseline or petroleum jelly since they can cause infection or irritation.

Urinary incontinence can occur from a weak PC (pubococcygeus) muscle. The "love muscle" is exercised by sexual intercourse or by squeezing the vagina as though trying to stop the flow of urine. It requires daily use - at least 200 contractions per day. Do 20 squeezes 10 times a day (at home, office, watching TV, etc.) Squeeze and relax the muscle as rapidly as you can and end with a long, sustained contraction. According to Dr. Kegel, these exercises have replaced the need for surgery in most women. It also helps to increase the intensity of orgasm. Men can also exercise their PC muscle and improve the pleasure and sensitivity of their orgasm.

Hot flashes can be reduced by exercise, which stimulates the ability to perspire and cools the body. The low-fat diet also may reduce symptoms and discomfort as your circulation improves. Consistent, vigorous exercise increases the circulation of both estrogen and adrenaline, toning the skin and muscles.

**Herbs, spices** and foods (over 150 herbs) for menopause were tested for effectiveness and reported results *Pro Soc Exp Biol Med 217, 1998.* Soy, licorice, red clover, thyme, turmeric, hops, and verbena helped modify estrogen activity the most. Oregano, verbena, turmeric, thyme, red clover and damiana balanced progesterone activity.

**Black cohosh** provided more relief from anxiety, depression, vaginal atrophy, hot flashes, headaches, dizziness, ringing in the ears, perspiration, palpitations, and sleep disturbances as compared to prescription drugs like valium and conjugated synthetic estrogen according to *Planta Medica 57, 1991, Med Welt 36, 1985, Theripeuticon 1:23, 1987, and Gyne 1:14, 1982.*

**Chaste berry** after 3 months daily capsule (20 mg) reduced prolactin release and estrogen production increased (*Arzneimittelforschung 43, 1993*). This is of benefit to menopausal women.

**Kava** worked better than tranquilizers in one week to reduce depression and improve feelings of well-being. It produces a feeling of happiness, more fluent lively speech, and sound sensitivity (*Pharmacopsychiatry 30, 1997*).

**St John's Wort** was found to be effective compared to placebo or antidepressants within 2 to 4 weeks to elevate mood, and reduce anxiety, depression.

**Gingko Biloba** – helps poor circulation to the brain, hands, legs, and feet (*Lancet 340, 1992*). It improves memory and slows dementia within 12 weeks or less (*JAMA 278, 1997*).

---

**Thyroid** is another anti aging hormone to monitor. If your thyroid level is low try taking supplements of glandulars, desiccated thyroid, (1/4 – grain per serving) or Armour. This is a natural form providing T3 and T4 that is more like that which the thyroid gland produces. People will feel better on it. Also be sure to use kelp for the iodine necessary for thyroid metabolism.

For years doctors have known that if a person has a low thyroid that he should have that thyroid level replaced. I don't think that there is a doctor in the country that would argue this and yet for various reasons some doctors are reluctant to understand the great advantage to replacing natural human growth hormone, DHEA, melatonin, and other associated hormones that are so critical. We have learned that progesterone improves thyroid activity.

When my partner Shawna started taking a natural thyroid replacement (thyroplex, and herbs-Black Walnut, Norwegian Kelp). I remember very distinctly that in a matter of a few days some of the changes that I noted were a change in her body temperature. Her hands always seemed to be cold even in rather warm weather and she became a rather hot bodied person. She formerly was very embarrassed to shake anyone's hand because her hands were always so cold. On particularly cold days she would become almost immobilized. The natural thyroid replacement worked wonderfully for her. She has also noted that if she runs out of her supply her levels start to decline again.

Thyroid & Thyroid Stimulating Hormone TSH benefits include:

- Improved sex drive, energy, less fatigue, and stronger
- Less colds, viruses, respiratory ailments, better breathing
- Warm hands & feet, stronger heart pump action
- Less muscle cramps, reduced low back pain, stiff joints, arthritis
- Prevent bruising, less dry skin & leathery skin; avoid brittle nails, hair loss.
- Ideal thyroid levels help mental acuity, improve memory, less emotional crying, upset
- Reduce Atherosclerosis, less headaches

A startling experiment on anti-aging demonstrated the power of **melatonin,** the actual hormone that controls the aging clock. The scientists transplanted the pineal gland from old mice into the young mice. They took the pineal gland from the young mice and transplanted it into the old mice. Melatonin is released in smaller quantities from the pineal gland as we age. The transformation was incredible! The older mice looked younger, with rejuvenated bodies. They were more active with a 30% extension in life span. The young mice with the old pineal gland aged rapidly and died 30% sooner than normal. The aging clock had finally unlocked the mysterious mechanism that determines not only how we age but also why we age.

The pineal gland in humans also sends out a message through melatonin to preserve the organs and the body in a healthy state. As we age, we must replace the dwindling melatonin to continue to preserve youth. It's best to take very small amounts of melatonin of one-tenth to one half mg (up to five mg) a night sublingual, dissolved under the tongue before you go to sleep. Increase gradually, so that you awaken in the morning alert and rested. If you awaken groggy, reduce the dosage back down by one half-milligram increment. Melatonin acts like a natural sleeping pill, enhancing REM dream sleep. Melatonin reduces jet lag, and resets the biological clock.

In a marriage, day people and night people can learn to match their schedule using melatonin. The person that tends to stay up late can take Melatonin at the time their spouse wants to go to sleep.

Melatonin has other benefits, according to the *New England Journal of Medicine, January 16,1997*. It is a free radical scavenger serving as an antioxidant inside the cells. It lowers cholesterol, heart disease, and cataracts. It may help Parkinson's disease, Alzheimer's and asthma and keep you young, vigorous and sexually rejuvenated.

Some people get worried that if they take hormone replacements that it will shut down their own body systems production. However, by augmenting and replacing that level that has declined due to aging, we are restoring it to a more youthful level. At youthful levels, we gain the benefit from natural and ideal levels of hormone replacement. If people stop taking the therapy after three months, they don't immediately revert back to a lower level compared to levels prior to therapy. The benefits they gained from the biochemical hormones remain for several weeks or months. However, without the supplements you will begin to notice the differences. Our brain and neural systems contain enzymes and steroid precursors such as cholesterol to convert into a variety of over 150 steroid and neurosteroid hormones. Scientists are still discovering new biochemical hormones that are created from the eight critical hormones.

William Regelson MD, age 71, has been taking DHEA everyday and one-tenth of a milligram of melatonin every night for eleven years. "I feel the difference. We need to treat aging as a disease, not just an irreversible condition." Dr. Regelson is a researcher at the Medical College of Virginia in Richmond.

Dr. Cranton MD told the story of a man age 72 years old who felt as if his life was winding down. He had no energy, reduced muscle tone, and he was falling asleep while driving. After eight months of hormone replacement he no longer needs as much sleep and he does not fall asleep while driving. The muscles in his legs and arms are strong and hardening. Now he runs up the steps in his house "as if I were twenty years younger. I thought my life was almost over, but now I'm planning to go to one hundred."

Now that you have learned about the latest research on anti-aging and hormone replacement let's not forget the important principals of healthy eating. People who want to look and feel great will do the following. I encourage the use of whole food concentrates, antioxidant's vitamin A, E,

C, B complex and whole food origins for minerals. Eat as much raw food as possible in the form of vegetables, fruit, sprouted seeds, sprouted beans and sprouted grains. I use a Vita-mix whole food machine or a simple blender to blend whole vegetables and fruit, retaining the fiber and all the vitamins, minerals and organic pure water. Use gluten and soy replacements for meat and rice milk for dairy product substitutes. Frequently nibble small meals, whenever you feel empty or hungry.

Exercise and activity has also been proven to reverse and slow aging. By following the Healthy Aging hormone replacement program you will have more energy to be able to workout with weights and do aerobics at least three times a week. Be physical and active. Enjoy holding, hugs, kisses and intimacy. Physical activity and intimacy will also increase your natural hormone production.

What can you expect from the Healthy Aging program? After only nine days most people will notice an improvement in energy levels, mental abilities, sleep habits, and sexual energy. After 90 days the fat on your body will begin to melt away using only natural approaches to enhance your body's proper metabolic levels. Your new Fountain of Youth habits will allow you to look and feel years younger. Your family and friends will notice the transformation and ask you what you have done.

## Nick Delgado Healthy Aging Hormone Fountain of Youth cocktail

1. Human Growth Hormone (HGH) – oral -use morning mid day and night
2. IFG-1 –oral morning, midday, and night
3. Preg- cream, sublingual, or capsules 2 mg to 15 mg in morning
4. DHEA – 2 mg to 15 mg – cream, sublingual or capsule –in morning
5. Melatonin- .1 to 1 mg sublingual- evening
6. Free Testosterone releasers: Avena Sativa- Green Oats, Nettle, Saw Palmetto niacin – men and women over age 35 – use daily
7. Total Testosterone for men increase ionic minerals with Zinc, Tribulus Terrestris fruit, Androstenedione or prescription testosterone gel micronized (micronized is a process that creates tiny particles for better absorption into the lymphatic system of the digestive tract to reduce liver breakdown in bloodstream)
8. Thyroid- Kelp, sea veggies/ thyroid glandulars (1/4 grain per serving)
9. Progesterone- Edens Secret or Pro-gest cream (men if poor bone density, women PMS, bone, youth)
10. Estrogen- black cohosh, phytogen, cayenne, noni, Es-Gen cream (women only) or prescription Triple or Bi Estrogen.

# III

# The Power of Blending & Sprouting, *Live* Enzymes, Phytochemicals, and Antioxidants for Energy

Wouldn't you like to perform at your absolute best always?

Athletes, sales people, children, housewives, and senior citizens can reach their peak potential and enjoy life more fully by eating more raw, sprouted, uncooked food, enzymes, herbs, hormones and exercising. The Peak performance plan requires a degree of discipline, commonly found in high achievers. Many people choose the immediate gratification of eating sweets and fats (short term goals of taste). Successful people have experienced the sweet rewards of security and happiness that comes with ideal health.

Successful people choose more healthful food selections and exercise to reach their long-term goals. They will bypass the temporary pleasure of sweets and select the foods necessary for performance at peak levels. Feeling good and looking great is a powerful motivation for health conscious people, isn't it?

People who value health, will exercise their bodies and minds daily to be as sharp as possible. Commit to 30 minutes of daily exercise and one hour of reading a night. You might make the excuse that "you don't have the time to exercise or to read" when in reality you do. Studies show that watching television dominates most free time. Yes, that means the three to eight hours of television that most people watch every day can be allocated to more productive pursuits. If you must watch television, then exercise aerobically on a reclined bike, Stairmaster, or treadmill while you watch. Better yet, consider reading while you exercise. You can be a wonderful role model for your children.

Here is the first key **dietary principle** to follow for **peak performance**:
Consume foods rich in complex carbohydrates in the raw state. Raw foods, such as fruit, vegetables, sprouted grains, sprouted legumes, and sprouted seeds are rich in digestive enzymes. The moment you heat the food by any method (lightly steaming, microwave oven, or stove) you destroy all the digestive enzymes in the food. Whole foods are rich in phytochemicals.

**PHYTOCHEMICALS** are naturally occurring chemicals in plants. Researchers have discovered over 103,000 phytochemicals. Some phytochemicals are anti-inflammatory, antibacterial, antiviral, and serve as an antioxidant able to capture free radicals and prevent them from damaging DNA. These protective phytochemicals appear to prevent the promotion of the carcinogenic process in two ways. First by acting as antioxidants that detoxify and block carcinogenic agents from reaching and penetrating cell bodies, and secondly, by increasing production and activity of enzymes that can suppress the expression of malignant changes in cells that have already been exposed and damaged by carcinogens. This may help reduce the incidence of breast, prostate, and colorectal cancers.

Other health benefits of phytochemicals include lowering cholesterol, detoxifying the liver, clearing-up bronchitis and nasal congestion, alleviating pain, healing stomach ulcers and stopping cramps. They can lower the number of histamines in the blood, which in turn reduces allergic reactions.

Supplements are available that contain components of whole, organic vegetable and fruit. The organic vegetables and fruit are harvested at the peak of maturity, when they are full of all the rich enzymes, minerals and phytochemicals. You should be able to break open a capsule and smell fresh fruit and vegetables. They can contain fresh spinach, lettuce, radish, carrot, beet, cabbage, celery, garlic, parsley, onion, nopal, broccoli, tomato, or apple, guava, grape, pear, watermelon, orange, pineapple, noni, peach, papaya and mango. Just two capsules have been estimated to contain the nutrients of one eight ounce glass of raw, fresh-squeezed juice.

Twenty-five percent of modern prescription drugs are artificial imitations of phytochemicals from plants. For example, the drug Taxol is an extract from the yew tree, used to treat ovarian cancer. This single drug will gross drug companies one billion dollars by the year 2000.

It is best to go to the source of whole food. Any disruption of the balance of whole food by juice extraction, peeling, degermination, and processing, reduces the healing powers and nourishing qualities of whole food sprouts, vegetables, fruit, beans, and grains.

An apple has only 12 vitamins and 13 minerals, however a whole apple also contains over 386 health-promoting phytochemicals that serve as cell protectors and detoxifiers. Squeezing the juice from an apple destroys much of its detoxifying, nourishing powers, because the apple pulp containing most of the value is discarded during juicing. Whole blended juice avoids this loss.

Extracted juices have a high concentration of sugar, which is absorbed too quickly into the bloodstream causing hyperglycemia, and release of insulin to store excess calories as fat. Whole blended juice avoids this problem. You'll notice a big difference when you drink whole blended juice or eat whole vegetables and fruit. You will feel satisfied and energetic, instead of hungry and weak with juice.

Drinking extracted juice leaves out most of the phytochemicals. Carrot juice has been considered beneficial because of beta-carotene. However, beta-carotene is just one of 500 carotenoids found in whole vegetables. Throwing away carrot pulp eliminates most of the powerful carotenoids that protect body cells and organs in a way that beta-carotene alone can not. It is possible that a high intake of just beta-carotene may impair the absorption of the other carotenoids. That could explain why a recent Finnish trail failed to prevent lung cancer using only beta-carotene.

Removing the pulp from carrots reduces our calcium intake by over 91%, your potassium by 50% and your magnesium by 69%. This decrease in available minerals can increase the risk of osteoporosis, allergies, and depressed immune function. The whole carotenoids enhance cell communication between pre-malignant and normal cells. Cell communication is how a healthy immune system is warned of intruders and in turn calls the body's defenses into action.

**Raw vegetable** whole *blended* juices, *blended* **sprouts**, and whole **fruit** juices can provide the richest source of organic water, fiber, phytochemicals, antioxidants, vitamins, minerals, and enzymes. **Do NOT use a juicer!** Buy a **simple blender** for under $99. The "best blender" is a *Vitamix* or *Bosch*, which is an investment in the $400 range. Is your health worth it? I believe it is, and the savings on using the blender instead of your juicer in wasting less volume of food and in health care costs are enormous. Other department store blenders work, they just have a smaller blender pitcher and a weaker motor. You may have to blend two batches instead of one batch. Most centrifugal force blenders create heat that can destroy some enzymes. You can add ice cubes and extra water during blending to keep the food cool, preserve enzymes and reduce the thickness to a drinkable liquid. The blender has a special motor that actually blends and retains all the fiber. Regular juicers discard all the essential fiber.

My recipes are different almost every morning or noon time. A typical blended drink might include sprouted sesame seeds, sprouted sunflower seeds, sprouted flaxseed, sprouted beans, sprouted grains with two carrots, one vine ripe tomato, one apple, blueberries, strawberries, and a banana. If it comes out too thick, I add rice milk or water to thin it out so I can drink the live blend of food. I keep fresh sprouts growing daily in four jars I rinse with water twice daily. The sprouts are ready in three to four days. If you don't have time to grow sprouts, you can buy sprout mixes at the market. The strong taste of sprouts is made palatable by the fresh fruit and carrots I add to this recipe. This makes about 64 ounces of blended thick juice for my family and me every morning. I notice I am not hungry for hours after drinking this wonderful life preserving drink. I have convinced hundreds of people to start blending instead of juicing, and every one of them has noticed a huge difference.

I mix in minerals from the oceans of *The Sea of Cortez*. According to Jacque Cousteau, it is pollution-free and "offers the most exciting array of marine species in the world." Another good source of **ionic minerals** comes from the coast of Hawaii. All **92** of the naturally occurring elements found in the seawater are also present in human tissues. I add these bioavailable trace minerals to my blended drink at least three times a week or more.

My son Nicholas and my daughter Cherish, enjoy their blended drinks with minerals. I find that to keep the drink palatable for them we have to include a higher percentage of fruits and vegetables with less sprouts.

Fruits and vegetables for breakfast, lunch, dinner, and snacks provide the purest source of fresh organic water, minerals, vitamins, fiber, and enzymes. You should consume over 10 servings of vegetables, sprouted grains, sprouted beans, sprouted seeds, and fruit. Within nine days you will feel the energy and power.

For a rich supply of enzymes, organic vitamins, and minerals, add to your lunch, dinner, or late meals a big bowl of raw vegetables with fat -- free dressing. Have sprouted sesame seeds, sprouted sunflower seeds, sprouted garbanzo beans, sprouted peas, sprouted bean mix, tomatoes, raw celery, carrots, broccoli, etc. We need a constant supply of fresh foods to get enough enzymes and antioxidants.

**ANTIOXIDANTS** such as Proanthocyanidins found in grapes are several times more effective than vitamin E and Vitamin C in protecting the body from the effects of free radicals. Increasing the intake of these antioxidants results in increased support of the immune system, assistance in collagen development and combating the aging of skin. Italian red grape seed contain a rich source of "Proanthocyanidins". Whole fruit and supplements are now available which contain citrus bioflavonoids, like quecitin, hesperidin, and rutin. The Peruvian herb Cat's Claw is another rich source of antioxidants and immune system booster. Oligomeric Proanthocyanidins (OPC) are another powerful antioxidant.

**ENZYMES** are essential to all of life's processes. If you deplete your enzyme supply you may weaken your immune system (increasing the risk of disease) and create malfunctions of other bodily systems such as your nervous system, respiratory, musculature, and skeletal systems. This can shorten your life span by as much as twenty years, according to Dr.

Edward Howell.

There are three ways to deplete our bodies supply of natural enzymes. One way to deplete our enzyme supply is by eating processed sugars, fats, and proteins. Sugars, fats, and proteins completely lack enzymes. They require excessive amounts of enzymes from the pancreas, stomach, and liver to complete digestion.

The second way to deplete our supply of enzymes is to eat too many cooked foods. The mildest form of heating food (over 118 degrees F) destroys all enzymes in the food. Lightly steamed, stir-fired, microwave or stove cooked destroy enzymes. A temperature that would be uncomfortable to the skin on your hand will destroy enzymes. Pasteurization is carried out at 145 degrees F. Water boils at 212 degrees F. Most cooking is carried out at 300 degrees F. or hotter!

The last way to deplete our enzymes is by consuming raw seeds, or raw nuts that have not been sprouted. Raw food that has not been sprouted contains enzyme inhibitors. Avoid enzyme inhibitors in raw foods (raw seeds, raw nuts, raw grains, or raw legumes), because they destroy your bodies limited supply of enzymes. Chickens and rats fed raw soybeans not sprouted or cooked become sickened and fail to grow. If you do eat any of these foods, be sure to sprout them. Sprouting the raw seed gets rid of enzyme inhibitors. Remember, legumes (beans) and grains are actually seeds before they are sprouted.

Another way to get rid of enzyme inhibitors in seeds is to cook the seeds. This is the only condition that we should cook any food. Nature provides enzyme inhibitors in seeds, nuts, grains, and legumes to prevent premature growth until being planted in a proper place. Seeds thousands of years old found in pyramids, still contain enzyme inhibitors. These enzyme inhibitors serve a vital role in preserving the plant species. Seeds that are extremely old, will sprout and grow within twenty-four hours after being planted in moist soil. The water soaks into the seeds, nuts, legumes, or grains and completely deactivates the enzyme inhibitors within twenty-four hours.

Start sprouting seeds, beans, peas, wheat, sunflower seeds, alfalfa seeds, lentils and chickpeas. Sprouting helps reduce the fat content of the seeds. It also enhances the protein and enzyme quality of the food so it is fresh and alive. *Live* food may include certain necessary nutrients we have yet to understand fully.

**Sprouting** is simple - place a teaspoon up to a quarter cup of seeds into a glass jar. It's best to use glass instead of plastic because the light coming through the glass affects the growth beneficially. A wire screen or a cheesecloth cover, works well. Add water and let the seeds soak overnight. Pour off the water the next day. Then, rinse the seeds with fresh water once or twice a day, perhaps in the morning and again at night. Leave the jar at a 45 degree angle after you pour out the water. Keep it in a dark area or in indirect light, since the sprouts grow best in this situation. Sprouts are ready to eat by the fourth day. Usually you can start a new jar one day, start another one the next and so on, for a constant supply of fresh sprouts. They're great for stuffing in sandwiches and salads. Sprouting can increase vitamin and mineral content of the food from fifty to nearly two thousand percent, especially for many B complex vitamins and vitamin C.

After three days, the sprouts are now little plants fully concentrated in beneficial enzymes. These digestive enzymes inside vegetables, fruits, sprouted wheat berries, or bean sprouts help our bodies during digestion. Without these plant enzymes, our bodies must draw on our own limited supply of enzymes to digest the food. Also, our body will convert some metabolic enzymes to be used as digestive enzymes. Eating cooked food can dangerously deplete our vital metabolic enzymes.

We have over 1,300 types of enzymes used in every bodily process. We have enzymes in every cell of our body; in our lungs, arteries, brain, and muscles to produce rapid chemical reactions so we can breathe, move, and even, think! The ability to think requires several chemical reactions initiated by enzymes. The only difference between life and death of a cell, tissue, or system is the presence of enzymes. Enzymes provide the actual God given spark of life, the vital living force within each of us. Enzymes are biologically active proteins that we are born with. We have a finite, limited supply of enzymes and when we run out or become too low in enzymes we become ill or die.

The same process of life or death occurs in all other animals and plants. The genetic clock is present in all animals, influenced by hormone levels, enzymes, and a coded gene for life and death. Death occurs after the gene sends a hormone signal to stop enzyme activity. To extend life to our full genetic capability, we must preserve and protect our enzymes.

Every time we eat junk food, cooked, processed, without enzymes, we deplete more of our storage of enzymes. The normal process of digestion uses up some of our digestive enzymes (lipase, protease, and amylase) in the mouth, stomach, and intestines. We rapidly deplete our storage of enzymes by eating highly processed sugars and fats. Still, the average American consumes over 130 pounds of sugar per year from soda pop, candy, and packaged foods. We consume more than 100 pounds of excess fat, and concentrated protein from cheese, meat, and oils.

It is no wonder that our body, designed to live over 120 years of life, barely makes it through 70 or 80 years of life. Animals fed cooked meat, seeds not sprouted, and processed foods (fatty or sugary) die prematurely. The same species of animal in captivity fed raw meat, or raw organic vegetables, and sprouts live a much longer life.

When I refer to organic, I am not talking about pesticide free (foods free of pesticides and additives are important for a different reason- to avoid toxins). **Organic food** is enhanced by living organisms such as plants and microorganisms. *Living* food converts all the vitamins, minerals, and nutrients into organic substances. **Organic** minerals, vitamins, and water are superior to **inorganic** sources. Organic water in fruits and vegetables contain organic minerals chemically improved by living organisms.

Plain tap or bottled water has an inferior source of minerals in the inorganic form. The only time you should consume additional bottled water, is just before an exercise session. Ideally, most of your water supply should come from whole fruits and vegetables, because it is **organic water** containing organic minerals. Organic, colloidal minerals are better because they are smaller and have an electrical charge. Inorganic minerals are too large to be used by the human body.

Most people take supplements of inorganic iron, sodium, or potassium from rock or nonliving substances produced by chemical reactions or man-made extractions. Synthetic, man-made vitamin C, Ascorbic Acid, lacks the beneficial properties of organic vitamin C bioflavonoids found in living, natural foods. The Ascorbic Acid is simply the outer-coating surrounding the essential bioflavonoids.

The organic sodium and potassium in celery are beneficial to our bodies enhancing enzyme activity and detoxification. Yet the sodium and potassium we get in table salt are potentially toxic to our bodies, blood pressure, heart rate, and enzyme activities. The organic iron in beet juice, green vegetables, and apples (there is more iron in the tart apple varieties like Granny Smith as compared to sweet red delicious) enhances red blood cell development. Yet the inorganic iron (ferrous sulfate) in supplement pills destroys hemoglobin and is potentially toxic to the liver (inorganic iron overload from pans or pills can cause death).

The "best supplement line" we recommend come from **whole plant foods** with capsules of concentrated raw vegetables, carrots, broccoli, grains and fruits. Capsules prepared without being heated are best. This preserves the enzymes, vitamins and minerals.

If you choose to eat cooked food, you should eat mostly whole, natural vegetarian food. The best grains to use in the cooked form would include: rice, rice pasta, rice cereals, rice milk ( Rice Dream) etc. Rice grains are best since they are the least allergic producing grains for most people.

Other good grains low in allergy properties would include kamut, spelt, or corn grains. These grains are less allergic producing then gluten containing grains so try them and monitor how you feel. Spelt, spelt bread, spelt pasta, spelt cereals (an ancient wheat free of gluten) are available in the health food store. Corn, corn flakes, corn tortillas are also good choices for an allergy free plan.

Cooking any of the above grains into bread will cause a complete loss of enzymes in the food, but it will get rid of the enzyme inhibitors. It is best to consume grains of any type after being sprouted. Fermenting of grains or soybeans is another way to get a rich source of enzymes. Fermented, predigested foods such as tofu (select the low-fat version), miso, and Tempeh are free of enzyme inhibitors, and are rich in good enzymes (if uncooked).

Add **digestive enzymes** from a plant source supplement sprinkled from ule into your food whenever you eat cooked foods. This will ; the loss of your limited supply of enzymes. Get an enzyme supp... lent that contains amylase (digests starch), protease (digest's protein), lipase (digests fat), sucrase and maltase (digest sugar). Open the capsule and sprinkle it on the cooked foods you eat. Sprinkling enzymes onto the food will allow the digestive process to begin immediately in the mouth and stomach. The addition of these supplements will help to preserve your enzymes. Be sure to select the capsules without bile. Bile is foul tasting. You should swallow and not break open capsules with bile.

Have you ever had constant, terrifying nightmares? I remember only too vividly, waking up in the middle of the night drenched in sweat, as I struggled to get away from some ominous fate. Looking back on those episodes, nightmares can be caused from eating too much meat (concentrated in fat and cooked protein) and dairy products (high in fat and pasteurized cooked protein). All of which can deplete enzyme levels and vitamin B6 and B complex.

A healthy individual should experience dream recall. If you cannot recall "good dreams", and you only remember nightmares (You wake fearful, worried, upset, death thoughts), you may be deficient in Vitamin B6. A good source of B6 is brown rice, bananas, corn, and carrot juice. Take a supplement of B6 of 100 to 600 milligrams per day until dream recall begins to occur, then taper off the dosage down to 2 to 25 mg per day. According to Carl C. Pfeiffer, Ph.D., MD, in his book *Nutrition and Mental Illness* a health practitioner may have you use a maximum of 2,000 mgs. per day until you experience dream recall. If you awaken every two hours during the night with vivid dreams, and remember up to four dreams in the morning you are getting too much B6. If B6 produces numbness of fingers or toes, shift to pyridoxal phosphate B6 at 200 mg.

For good mental health avoid being contaminated with copper from birth control pills, drinking water from copper pipes, or any supplement with added copper. Use other forms of birth control such as condoms. Use filtered water, and get most of your water from fruits and vegetables. When I'm thirsty, the first thing I eat is a juicy tomato, or grapes.

What if you have been exposed to any of the above sources of concentrated copper? Check with a doctor to have your copper levels and zinc levels in the urine, blood plasma and hair measured. If copper is found to be elevated and zinc low, take the antidote of zinc gluconate, 15 mg to 30 mg a day. Also you should consume more tropical fruits like mangos and pineapples for a source of manganese. Zinc can cause an imbalance in manganese, this is why you need to add manganese when taking zinc supplements. Manganese gluconate of 10 to 50 mg a day will prevent any problems.

Some conditions that have been helped by treating high copper levels, added zinc and manganese include:
Paranoia, disperceptions, feelings of persecution, fearful-feelings, Autism, loss of contact with reality, schizophrenia (a misleading
Diagnosis or false label), depression, anemia compulsions, hallucinations, impotence, and nervous exhaustion.

Additional tests your doctor might run include blood and urine histamines levels. Also, check the blood for vitamin B6. You should have your cholesterol level done as part of a lipid panel, a chemistry panel with liver and kidney enzyme levels, and CBC with blood morphology.

Your brain will function best with ideal blood glucose levels (the brain can only use glucose for fuel). To prevent hypoglycemia (low blood sugar), eat frequent small meals of fresh fruits, vegetables, sprouted peas, and rice based products. Carry a cool tote and frozen blue ice, filled with fruits and vegetables, with you always. Take fresh food with you to the office and on the road. Nibble the moment you are hungry. Eat every few hours, or every twenty minutes if need be. Anticipate your hunger and eat if you feel weak or empty. The results will be tremendous within a short period of time.

Our studies show that the average person with an elevated cholesterol level can reduce it by as much as 30% by dietary changes alone. You can reduce and control triglyceride (fat in the blood) by as much as 40% within nine days (with added exercise). Improved circulation will do wonders for your performance, sense of well being, and energy levels.

I modified my diet using the Juice blend recipe in the morning to include additional sprouts, fruits and vegetables above my normally high raw food intake. After only six months, I noticed increases in energy, less body fat and gain's of lean body muscle mass. This brought me to ideal levels as if I was twenty years younger. I have placed first and second in the best body contest "Mr. Mastery" at the Anthony Robbins event in La Jolla, California 1992 and Cancun, Mexico 1993. I live each day feeling and looking in the peak of health. How about you? Are you ready to experience a whole feeling of wellness?

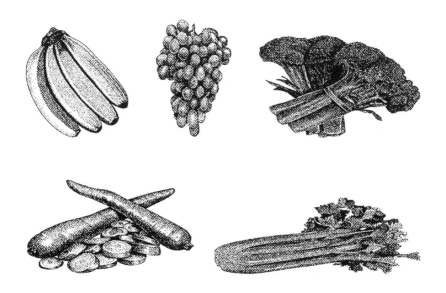

# IV

∞

# Herbs are Plants used as Medicine

For centuries people have used herbs because of their pleasing smell or taste, and for medicinal purposes. The use of herbs in healing the sick has survived for countless years because herbs are organic and therefore, are capable of becoming a part of the living organism. They are the source and origin of all life on earth. The herb assimilates inorganic mineral matter and convert it into living organic material, which when presented to the animal or human cell, is absorbed, renewing and sustaining its life process.

We have identified over 380,000 species of plants on earth and several hundred thousand that have yet to be discovered! Nearly 260,000 plants are classified as higher plants, because they contain chlorophyll to perform photosynthesis. Only 26,000 plants in this group are studied and used for health benefits. However, over 230,000 plants may provide benefits, yet scientists are trying to catalogue these plants as potential plant cures. Unfortunately, certain areas like the Amazon rainforest are being destroyed and many plant species may never be studied.

In the United States, herbs are not recognized as drugs, and labeling cannot offer therapeutic advice. Your pharmacist and most doctors rarely have taken a course in pharmacology on herbs. Drug companies have begun to look into herbs, however patents are not issued for natural herbs and studies are not performed. I have read and studied about herbal medicine and I'm convinced this natural approach will continue to flourish.

Herbs offer powerful rejuvenating qualities. Science is now having a renewed interest in herbalism because they work. Just as nutrition and lifestyle play important roles in disease prevention, it is being shown that herbs can also play a significant role in promoting wellness. Studies show that herbs have been shown to reduce cholesterol, improve circulation, and even prevent cancer! Wouldn't we all prefer to take an herb to stay healthy than a drug when we are sick. There are herbs that soothe pain and inflammation or that work to reduce muscle spasm. Some herbs kill bacteria, others activate the body's own immune system so that it can ward off invading organisms. And there are herbs that target specific organs.

Unfortunately there is a misconception that because herbs are "natural", they can be taken by chance. This is not the case! Herbs can be a strong medicine. It is best if people do not attempt to gather thier own herbs, because 1 percent of all plants are poisonous. Make sure you know how to use it and what it does to avoid any possible side effects. It is best to buy prepared herbal remedies from companies with standardized, uniform levels of the compound and guaranteed potency. Purchase fresh, freeze-dried herbs because they preserve more of the herb's active ingredients, organically grown and non-irradiated.

Hippocrates, the father of medicine wrote these words: "Let thy food be thy medicine and thy medicine be thy food." Around 390 BC he advocated the use of plant medicines and diet to prevent and cure diseases. The Hippocratic oath, do no harm,was based on teaching the power of using over 400 natural plant medicines. We have learned after thousands of years of using herbs that they work because of active ingredients that exert a profound effect on our tissues and organs. For example, foxglove is a fuchsia-flowered plant with glycosides that stimulate heart cells and treat heart failure. Comfrey leaf has the astringent tannins to promote healing of wounds. Licorice has sponins, an anti-inflammatory compound to soothe arthritic flare-ups. Garlic has volatile oils that fight infection.

It is usually best to take herbs after a meal, rather than on an empty stomach to avoid nausea that some people might experience. Start with the lowest dosage recommended on the label and work your way up to maximum dosage. If you experience relief at the lower dosage, there is no need to increase. Most herbs are taken for brief intervals to remedy various conditions. Animal behaviorists have observed many animals seek specific plants when they are sick. Early humans starting in India still practice Ayurveda medicine today. Sumerians used herbs over 5,000 years ago such as caraway and thyme for healing. Onions and garlic were favorites of the Egyptians. Over 3,000 years ago Chinese herbal medicine included ginger, astragalus root, and licorice. The bible is full of herb references such as aloe, myrrh, and frankincense. The famous physician, Galen (AD 137), blended herbs and cures for Roman emperors and gladiators.

Today, herbal medicine is still the primary source of health care for 80 percent of the world's population. The eighteenth century physician Samuel Hahnemann and other homeopathic physicians relied on drugs derived from plants or animals in their practice. Many western medical establishments are starting to consider alternatives to harsh drugs such as those used in chemotherapy.

Herbs can be a great way to assist you in fat loss. Herbs can make you feel more energy. When you have more energy, you feel like going out and doing things, going for walks, riding bicycles, and being outdoors. As you become more active you will lose more fat. Herbs also help to reduce appetite, helping you to eat smaller more frequent meals and only when you're hungry. As you lose pounds of fat, your energy level increases and your hunger urge decrease with herbs.

Herbs are available as capsules, tablets, powders, creams, ointments, extracts, or tinctures of liquid. Essential oils are used for external application. Herbal shampoos, facial cleansers, deodorants, moisturizers, toothpaste, and mouthwash, and cosmetic lines are excellent alternatives to chemical-laden, irritating products.

These are the top HERBS I have selected to give you the best benefits in alphabetical order. Obvious cautions to not use herbs during pregnancy, unless under doctors orders (typically because certain herbs can stimulate contractions etc., check with your doctor if your taking prescription drugs (because herbs can magnify results above expectations, and you may need to reduce dosages). If you experience any allergic reactions or unexpected side effects, have the PRIME test(read section on allergies in this book) for verification. Lastly, don't take herbs above the suggested usage (started with lowest amounts on labeled package) because they are powerful natural medicines. Please Reference *The Complete Medicinal Herbal* by Penelope Ody.

**Aloe Vera-** is mentioned in the Bible under PROVERBS 7:17. Aloe gel is regarded as one of nature's best natural moisturizers. Queen Cleopatra regarded the gel as a fountain of youth and used it to preserve her skin against the ravages of the Egyptian sun. Aloe effectively treats wounds, burns, skin abrasion. It's anti-fungal, stops bleeding, and acts as sedative.

**Alfalfa-**natural diuretic, laxative, boosts appetite, reduce cystitis.

**Astragalus-** activates the immune system to fight disease and cancer. It can reduce blood pressure because it rids the body of excess water weight, and it is a mild stimulant used in weight loss formulas.

**Bee Pollen-** contains 22 basic elements found in the human body, rich in vitamins, minerals, amino acids, hormones, enzymes, and essential fats helpful in slowing the aging process.

**Bilberry-** was given to Royal Air Force pilots during World War II to enhance night vision. It may even help near-sightedness. It is rich in proanthocyanins an effective antioxidant flavonoid.

**Black Cohosh-** American Indians used it for pain, inflammation of joints, and female cramps. It is used for persistent coughs of asthma, bronchitis, and whooping cough.

**Black Walnut-** useful against fungal and parasitic worm infections, warts, eczema, psoriasis, herpes, and skin rashes.

**Buchu-**Tribes in South Africa used this aromatic plant for urinary disorders like cystitis, urinary tract infections, prostate problems. It is a good diuretic to reduce excess water weight, bloating and it promotes perspiration. It has a stimulating effect on the body.

**Burdock-** purifies blood by increasing flow of urine and promotes sweating. Soothes pain of arthritis and backache. A natural diuretic to rid the body of excess water weight.

**Borage-** stimulates the adrenal gland for fight or flight to handle stress. This herb oil contains essential fatty acids( linoleic & gamma-linolenic acids), promotes lactation, sweating, relieves irritable bowel syndrome.

**Cascara Sagrada-**natural laxative, expel worms, parasites, help blood pressure, insomnia, gall stones, liver and gallbladder problems.

**Cat's Claw (Una de Gato)-** helps the immune system fight cancer, viruses, ulcers, and inflammation.

**Capsicum or Cayenne-** hot spicy peppers are incredible high in Vitamin C, A, B-complex, and calcium. They stimulate the production of gastric juices, relieve gas, improve metabolism, promote sweating, and increases blood flow. Used for headaches, arthritis, ulcers, and lower blood lipids.

**Cranberry-** herbs without added sugar prevent urinary infections by preventing bacteria from sticking to the wall of the bladder ridding the body of buildup.

**Devil's Claw-** promotes flexibility of joints, reducing pain of arthritis. It helps diabetes, kidney & liver problems, reduces lipids.

**Dong Quai-** used in Chinese medicine to reduce menstrual cramps, PMS, hot flashes, insomnia, anemia, and high blood pressure.

**Ecinacea-** enhances the immune system and prevents viruses and pathogens like herpes, colds, flu, candida fungus, eczema, and psoriasis.

**Ephedra (Ma Huang)-** has been used to treat asthma, colds, allergy symptoms and is considered a long acting stimulant used in many weight loss products.

**Evening primrose-** Native Americans used it as a painkiller because it's rich in essential oils to convert hormones of prostaglandins. It helps PMS, breast tenderness, bloating, anxiety and eczema of the skin-cradle cap in infants.

**Fennel Seed-** is used to relieve gas, stimulate appetite, expectorant for coughs and colds, and relieves joint stiffness due to arthritis.

**Flax or linseed oil-** soothing gastritis, sore throat, anti-inflammatory, diuretic, and antiseptic.

**Ginkgo biloba-** is used for coughs, asthma, and inflammations due to allergies. It increases blood flow to the extremities, inner ear, brain, and enhancing memory. It slows the aging process.

**Ginseng, Siberian-** enables the body to cope with stress, increase energy, improves estrogen normalization, & enhances sexual desire.

**Suma (Brazilian ginseng)-**energy tonic, for menopause, fatigue, stress.

**Golden Seal Root-** a treatment for gonorrhea, syphilis, colds, flu, candida fungus, ringworm, canker sores, ulcers, & vaginal infection.

**Gotu Kola-**promotes relaxation, enhances memory, and circulation.

**Guarana-** has been used in Brazil, and now the U.S. for increased mental alertness and to fight fatigue. It's popular in weight loss formulas. The seeds of the plant contain 5% caffeine and stimulates the body.

**Hawaiian Noni-**Islanders use it for pain, infections, fungus, parasites, PMS, to stimulate the immune system and conditions of aging.

**Hawthorn Berries-** relaxes peripheral blood vessels improves blood flow, rid body of excess salt and water.

**Juniper Berries-**is good for digestion and can eliminate gas, cramps, and urinary retention. It has been used for gout arthritis, gallstones, and it rids the body of excess fluid.

**Kava Kava**-is used for nervousness, stress, insomnia, promotes sleep, relieves cramps due to muscle spasms, and reduces water retention.

**Norwegian Kelp**- over 30 minerals including iodine for goiter- thyroid, helps acne, PMS, obesity and nervous disorders.

**Licorice**-detoxifies poisons, joint pain, congestion, ulcers, cancer.

**Marshmallow Root**-is high in mucilage, soothes ulcers, colitis, enteritis.

**Milk Thistle**- rejuvenates the liver, increases bile to break down fat.

**Myrrh**- removes bad breath, heals cold sores, fever blisters, herpes.

**Nettle**-for stuffy nose, allergy, vaginal infection, low blood sugar.

**Pau d' Arco**- for athlete's foot(fungal), parasitic infection, diabetes.

**Red Clover**-, for muscle relaxer and immune system.

**Saw Palmetto**- to reduce prostate enlargement, aphrodisiac, relieves chest congestion.

**Shiitake Mushroom**- immune system cancer fighting agent, cholesterol.

**St. John's Wort**- for wounds, depression, inflammation and cancer.

**Tea Tree Oil**- Chemical analysis of tea tree oil ( Melaleuca Alternifolia) Shows that the oil consists of 48 different compounds. Chemistry and pharmaceutical experts believe that a combination of all the oils compounds working together makes it effective. Terpinen 4-ol is know to be one of the most important therapeutical qualities in tea tree oil. Cincole is somewhat caustic and helps the oil to penetrate. Tea tree oils are soothing and also considered a natural analgesic. It can be a natural antiseptic, a natural germicide and bacteriacide. It doesn't destroy the living tissue, and allows the healthy tissue to heal together with little or no scarring. It is considered to be a natural fungicide killing fungus in all forms such as athlete's foot, mold and mildew and candida albicans. Tea tree oil's properties of cincole, allows the oil to penetrate through all the skin layers and into the muscle. It is a natural solvent and it is aromatic. It can be used in a spray bottle or in a vaporizer. For years, tea tree oils have been used as an enhancement to perfume.

**Uva Ursi**- is effective for bladder, kidney ailments, urinary tract infections. In weight loss programs it is used as a diuretic.

**Valerian**-lowers blood pressure, stress, anxiety, alcoholism & gas.

**Yerba Santa**- help cough, phlegm, allergy, hayfever, asthma.

**Yucca**- reduce inflammation of arthritis.

# V

∞

# The Key to Making Changes is Using Power Questions?

We have over 50,000 thoughts a day and a majority are negative, self-defeating thoughts like "I can't do this or that." What if you started replacing every negative thought with a positive question? Your brain is like a problem-solving computer that wants to come up with answers and solutions. Believe it or not, it will change your life! Every aspect of your life can be remolded and shaped to your desire by asking yourself the right types of questions. Take each aspect of your life that you want to improve starting with values that are most important to you. Start with health, love, wealth, happiness, growth, personal development, and any other area you want to improve upon.

I keep a written list of power questions with me to read from every morning or just before I go to sleep. I focus on what I want from life and I ask myself power questions to nurture positive thoughts and solution oriented actions.

It is very important you ask the right type of questions to get the best outcome. For example, in the area of health, if you think thoughts like "I'll never be able to lose this body fat" or "why am I so fat?" You're mind will think negative thoughts. You might mistakenly believe you're just undisciplined and it's genetic. This may cause a defeated attitude and lack of action while you gain more weight every year. It would be more effective to ask yourself "what exercise can I do today to reduce body fat?" Your brain will scan your memory banks for your favorite aerobic exercises! Here are some of the questions I ask myself everyday related to my values of health and life. You're welcome to use these as a guide if you want to be happier!

**Improving my health with better food and supplement selections**

Which raw vegetables, sprouts, seeds, beans, and fruit will I eat more of today? Did I have a morning, noon or evening blended raw vegetable, sprout, and fruit drink? How many salads or vegetable dishes could I enjoy eating today? Is my cool tote filled with my favorite fresh vegetables, fruit and supplements to take with me to work? Do I need to go to the produce store or health food store to restock my high-energy foods today?

Which supplements will I take today to cleanse my body, burn fat, build, rejuvenate and energize my body? Did I pack my supplement tray in my cool tote today?

How can I reduce fat, cholesterol, and sugar in my diet and make better choices dining out or at home? How can I avoid the consumption of animal products and what tasty substitutes can I consume? What foods rich in fiber will I eat more of today?

**Improving your fitness and energy level**

What actions and activities can I take part in today to raise my energy level? Is my gym bag ready with portable tape player, workout journal, and athletic shoes? It is best for me to workout in the morning, or have I scheduled time in the evening for a workout? Can I go dancing tonight? When can I go biking or participate in sports activities with the kids or friends? Did I get enough sleep and feel refreshed? Do I need to set time today for quiet time, mediation or a nap?

What is my current body fat level? Quarterly assessment for blood, saliva, urine test for ideal biochemical hormones-DHEA, IGF-1, Free testosterone, thyroid TSII, progesterone, estrogen, lipids, chemistries, blood cell quality, acid-alkaline balance, and free-radical damage?

**Emotional health, happiness & spirit**

Did I ask forgiveness and communicate with the Lord? Have I avoided spending too much time with stressful, negative people? What have I done today to strengthen my family to withstand confrontations? What successful people can I spend more time with this week for master minding and networking?

**Learning from failure is necessary to be successful**

What did I learn from my mistakes today? What will I do differently in future events to insure a better outcome? What or who have I avoided and what action can I take today to overcome my fears?

**Love, passion, sex, romance, companionship, friendship**

Did I spend quality time with my mate, family and friends today? Did I allow private time for romance with my lover tonight and satisfy her needs?

**Contributing to family and society**

In what ways can I contribute to the lives of those who have helped my family and me? What worthy cause or group can I donate time, knowledge or assistance? What activity do my children enjoy doing and have I scheduled time for those events? Have I shared or read stories of success and overcoming adversity with family or friends today?

**Personal development and growth**

What books, tapes, references, computer sources, or seminars can I learn from this week? What time have I spent today on major dreams or projects that will some day be a huge accomplishment? Have I taken time to consider what's important to my family, and me and what motivates each of us? Have I allowed time for entertainment and rewards for living according to my values?

**Wealth, prosperity, security**

What is the best use of my time right now? Who can I meet with this week to create or maintain business? What projects or vehicles can I invest in to create a better return for my time? What areas can I be more responsible about in my life or business relationships?

**Health & success require an honest appraisal of your life**

You must first make an honest appraisal of your current status regarding health and the quality of your life. This appraisal will help you to focus the appropriate time and energies needed to constantly improve. Those areas that are going well will require less effort. The areas you are weak in will require additional education, focus, discipline and changes of behavior. You must face the truth and the reality of the status of your life and health in order to change. If you accept being obese and out of shape, you will tend to make excuses for yourself and never make the effort or pursue solutions. Initially, it may be easier for you to cope with your physical inequities, however in order to be successful you must be honest with yourself. Otherwise, you will continue to delude yourself by thinking everything about your life is fine and there is no need to change.

How do you describe yourself - physically? Great, Good, fair, poor, or needing massive change? Given your current health habits or lack of, will you be in better, the same or worse health 10 years from now? Do you spend most of your time around people doing better than you do physically? Worse, or the same as you? What time wasters can you discard for a better use of your time with family, exercise, or career? TV, bars, reading or listening to negative news? What time can you schedule to consistently meet with a personal trainer, wellness mentor, or doctor? How much time and money can you invest each day or week in exercise, nutrition, supplements? How well do you understand the ill effects of over-consuming dairy, meat, chicken, sugar, salt, fat and alcohol?

Are you willing to eliminate the **negative beliefs** about health like: I have to starve to lose weight, I don't have time for exercise, exercise tires me out, disease happens for no reason, I'm helpless to prevent disease. My new **Positive beliefs** are frequent exercise and rest gives me more energy, power and vitality. Disease is a signal I need to make changes in my approach to health care. I choose to eat foods and take supplements that help me to reduce body fat, and increase my energy level. I can prevent slow or reverse diseases of aging. Have you had thorough tests to monitor premature aging? Hormonal, body fat, carotid artery scan for plaques in arteries, cholesterol, HDL, LDL, triglycerides?

Are you willing to consistently monitor your progress and correct when you're off course? You agree it is best to live a balanced life regarding health, vitality, happiness, career, and relationships don't you? How much would it be worth to you, your family and those you love, if you strive towards your values and goals? How soon will you take action to becoming healthier, happy, and vital- today, next week, in a month?

**Ask Bob Wieland if he knows the power of questions.** Bob is is a double amputee who nearly died in Vietnam after a bomb blew off his legs. He survived to become one of the great speakers and motivators of our time. I first met Bob in San Gabriel, California at the end of a seminar I was conducting in 1979 for over 300 people at the San Gabriel Community Hospital, when I worked as Director of the Pritikin Wellness plan with the famous, Nathan Pritikin.

Bob Wieland decided to ask a question if he could rebuild peoples' mental disabilities and lack of inspiration. I trained Bob to present our wellness seminars. I was and still am impressed with Mr. Wieland's courage and success-oriented attitude. His sharp mind and personal motivation has allowed him to exceed world records in the bench press. He has entered and competed against able-bodied athletes in the physically and mentally demanding, **Iron Man Triathlon** in Kona, Hawaii (26-mile run, 2.4 mile swim, and 112 mile bike race). At the *New York City Marathon*, I personally covered the course with Bob, taking all night into the next day (about 96 hours). This unbelievable, real life story doesn't just end here; instead of using a wheelchair, Bob covered the entire 26-mile course walking on his hands! Imagine starting in a seated position, he leans forward with his awesome upper body strength, planting his arms as a pivot for him to swing his trunk 3 feet at a time!

The next part of this true story sounds impossible and beyond imagination. Bob decided to walk across America on his hands, over 5 million steps, taking nearly four years! The greatest physical feet ever performed in my opinion. When asked how he did it? Bob's reply "one step at a time, but the hardest step of all was the first one." His decision to become great, and have an impact on other people, has impacted more young lives than any other speaker in the country. Bob as of this writing is 53 years old and in phenomenal shape physically and mentally.

Adversity and negativity doesn't exist in Bob Weiland's conversation or thoughts, only challenges to overcome. Bob takes supplements, trains in the gym, goes to church and prays that others will learn from his example. Bob and I have conducted hundreds of seminars together over the last twenty years. We believe that you were born to succeed. However, you have to take that first step and follow the *Healthy Aging Program*.

I met another great man, named Nathan Pritikin in 1978. He was 63 years old at the time and I was 23 years old. I was amazed by his energy and persistence compared to other men of his age. I worked as his right hand along side him (I become Director of the entire community based program). We developed a wellness program for a whole city in Louisiana. We started providing hospital wellness programs to train doctors about preventative health care. I did the first seminars with Nathan in San Diego, California at Kaisier Permanente Hospital for over 60 doctors, in 1982.

Nathan Pritikin was great researcher and a pioneer in wellness care. He had over 50 patents worldwide in chemistry, physics and electronics. Our Longevity program was featured on CBS's *60 minutes* with a record for viewer response. We documented our results and reported them in medical journals of reversing degenerative diseases. Famous authors, politicians, actors, and corporate presidents came to us to have their lives improved at our live-in centers and outpatient clinics. It only took four weeks to train people how to overcome even the most difficult of health problems. Nathan and I presented powerful seminars, documented by thousands of medical references that we had read. Pritikin and I answered difficult questions to the satisfaction of participants with serious diseased conditions, explaining complex issues that few doctors were able to understand. Nathan was a genius, and I will forever be grateful to him for having the opportunity to witness the development of today's Healthy Aging program. Our continued efforts have taught us many new things since those days. Hundreds of thousands of people have already benefited from this program that allows you to slow down aging and live a better quality life. You have the opportunity now to benefit from this powerfully effective anti-aging program.

This Healthy Aging approach can allow you reduce your risk of dying prematurely from diseases normally associated with aging including cancer, heart disease, stroke or diabetes. More important than living longer; you will feel more energy, look better than you have in years, quiet possibly than ever, and be able to cope better with the challenges we face on a daily basis. Apply the information today, keep track of your progress and send us an update of how you are doing. We promise to read every letter.

# VI

∞

# Amazing Supplements: Vitamins & Minerals

Food and supplements derived from organic food is the best source to meet your nutritional needs for vitamins, minerals and enzymes. Only 100 vitamins, minerals and nutrients have been discovered at this time, and the possibility remains several more will be found. Your best chance of obtaining the nutrition you need would be from whole natural foods like vegetables, fruits, grains, beans and sprouted seeds. Choose supplements derived from a variety of whole natural foods. Look closely upon labeling and ask if they are synthetic or chemically derived. The **label** must list actual whole food ingredients. I have only found a few companies that market this top of the line products.

There are advanced delivery systems to carry vitamins and minerals to your cells using **liposomes**, or tiny spheres made of soy lecithin. These multi-layered spheres are 1/50$^{th}$ the diameter of a human hair. They are able to deliver water soluble and fat-soluble vitamins, minerals, and nutrients. The liposomes penetrate the mucosal tissue of the mouth or skin and the nutrients are released from billions of liposomes suspended into the bloodstream. This path bypasses the digestive system longer. Stomach acids destroy many nutrients, and the nutrients are metabolized in the liver and broken down prematurely. Liposomes taken orally, or rubbed into the skin increase absorption of supplements, and act longer in the body enhancing bioavailability.

Supplements are available using ionic or *micro dispersions of supplements* in minute particles. Plants naturally draw nutrients up through roots like a filter and ionize or allow only microscopic size nutrients. Supplements with this delivery system are desirable because they are similar to what your body is accustomed to.

You may need to use supplements with our program, but only if you're eating processed foods, white flour, sugar or alcohol, or if you live in a polluted environment. Who doesn't have these situations? They are very common. In other words, we know you're going to cheat on occasion. You might want to take a vitamin-mineral supplement as a preventive formula. You want a multiple vitamin and mineral that at least meets the RDAs (possibly with more B complex, if you drink alcohol or get more sugar in your diet than you want). You need to understand safe ranges because too many supplements can be toxic. The following is a guideline of vitamins and minerals found in foods and their role in good nutrition.

I have found the best way to be consistent about taking my supplements is to carry with me a **SUPPLEMENT BOX** or utility container with several compartments for my various vitamins, minerals, enzymes, and herbs. The top natural bodybuilders like Skip LaCour have used a supplement container packed in his cool tote for convenience and frequent access.

Many nutritionists are trained by professors advocating the outdated four food groups and by textbooks (prepared from studies paid for by the meat and dairy industry). The use of liver, eggs, cheeses and meat is not good sources of vitamins and minerals because of the excess fat, protein and cholesterol content. Do not be misled into believing you need these harmful foods for "proper nutrition".

### VITAMIN A
This substance comes from either animal or vegetable sources. Vitamin A helps you maintain the quality of the mucous membranes and to resist infections. It is essential for bone growth, reproduction, white blood cell development and normal vision. It has some activity as an antioxidant, yet it works best with beta-carotene and up to 500 carotenoid. The animal source of Vitamin A is somewhat toxic. A deficiency of Vitamin A, however, has led to an eyeball disease, blindness of the eye and aged skin. We can avoid both problems, getting too much or too little, simply by relying on the vegetable source of Vitamin A, betacarotene and carotenoids, because you cannot overdose on the vegetable source.

For example, a cup of carrots has about 16,000 I.U. of Vitamin A, and a cup of sweet potatoes about 20,000 I.U. The Recommended Daily Allowance (RDA) is only about 5,000 I.U. Somewhere between 5,000 and 15,000 would meet anyone's needs.  If you ate too many carrots, sweet potatoes, mustard greens or squash, eventually your skin may turn a little orange or yellow. Once your body is ready to convert the betacarotene underneath the skin into Vitamin A, it will; there is no toxicity known with vegetables, so it is perfectly safe to take supplements derived from plant sources.  Yellow and orange-colored vegetables and fruit, such as cantaloupe, contain the good type of Vitamin A (beta-carotene & carotenoids).  Our Healthy Aging Plan supplies more than enough Vitamin A, and certainly more than the typical American diet.

We want you to avoid the animal sources of Vitamin A as much as possible.  Liver, egg yolks and butter fat are high sources of Vitamin A and can be toxic, especially if you take in 100,000 international units (I.U.) per day.  This sources of Vitamin A can build-up in your tissues and lead to side effects.  In a four month period, the animal source was shown to cause nerve, bone and cartilage damage.  It has been known to halt growth in children, lead to blurred vision, headaches, hair loss and to force cholesterol deposits into the tissues.

**Vitamin A**   RDA: 5,000 I.U.  If you use animal source supplement is up to 15,000 I.U.  Vegetable source supplements are your best choice.

| 1 CUP | I.U. |
| --- | --- |
| Hot, red chili peppers | 23,500 |
| Sweet potatoes, mashed | 20,150 |
| Carrots, cooked | 16,280 |
| Pumpkin, Collards, mustard greens | 16,000 to 14,760 |
| Butternut squash, Dandelion greens | 13,120 to 13,000 |
| Carrots, raw, nori seaweed | 12,100 to 11,000 |
| Garden cress, Kale, Turnip greens | 10,400 to 8,000 |
| Winter squash, mango (1/2) | 8,000 to 7,920 |
| Swiss chard, beet greens | 7,830 to 7,400 |
| Amaranth grain, Muskmelons, Parsley | 6,100 to 5,100 |
| Red bell peppers, cantaloupe, Broccoli | 4,450 to 3,880 |
| Apricots (3 average) | 2,890 |

## VITAMIN E
Vitamin E is important to prevent rancidity.  It helps the oxygen in the body and protects the cells.  Vitamin E is also necessary on a low-fat diet, however,

people following a high fat diet tend to require more. It is a good antioxidant, protecting you from free-radical pathology, heart disease, aging and cancer. Vitamin E improves the efficient use of oxygen and decreases platelet stickiness, which reduces excessive blood clotting, offering protection from sudden blockage of an artery. It works with other antioxidants and free-radical scavengers. Dietary essential fatty acids are also protected from oxidation with Vitamin E. When you take Vitamin E as a supplement, it's best not to exceed 400 I.U. You may have symptoms of fatigue using the oil based Vitamin E from increased rate of triglycerides (fat) in the blood.

It is true we need Vitamin E, and it would be best to take supplements derived from whole natural foods. For example, kale, cucumbers, or collards contain Vitamin E. Cucumbers contain about 8 I.U. per cup; two cups would complete your entire requirement for the day. Summer squash, millet, green peas and various other fruits and vegetables provide additional Vitamin E. Add a dry form (d-alpha tocopheryl Succinate, Beta, Gamma, Delta Tocopherols) sufficient to obtain Vitamin E.

**Vitamin E** RDA: 15 I.U. Best not to exceed 400 I.U./day. If you reduce fat in your diet, Vitamin E is used more efficiently.

| 1 CUP | I.U. |
|---|---|
| Collards, Cucumbers, Kale, Summer Squash | 15.00 to 7.5 |
| Millet, Turnip greens, Whole wheat flour | 4.00 to 3.12 |
| Green peas, Asparagus, Herring, Hazelnuts(6) | 3.00 to 1.80 |
| Mango (1/2), Almonds (6), whole wheat bread (3) | 1.50 t0 1.00 |
| Banana, Leeks, Chestnuts, mushrooms, Celery | 1.00 to .57 |
| Tomato, Onions, Grapefruit | .54 to .26 |

## VITAMIN B-12

B-12 is part of the B complex family and is necessary to good health. The B complex vitamins help your body to use carbohydrates, to burn them for energy and to use the protein and the fat you eat. Vitamins should not be taken without food because they are like an enzyme that helps to put the food to use. Some people fast or skip meals and then take vitamins believing they're helping themselves. When you do take vitamin supplements, you should take them with your food, and you should depend on your food as your primary nutrient source.

Vitamin B-12 deficiencies could result in pernicious anemia. Only a few cases of dietary B-12 deficiencies have been reported in scientific literature, and those cases were associated with intestinal disorders. If there was an absorption problem, there would be an intrinsic factor enzyme that would be absent because of a disease of the stomach or small intestines. In that event, although you were getting enough B-12, you may not be able to absorb it and you may need an injection once every three months. Equally effective, according to the British Medical Journal (291:56,1985), would be one large daily dose, 1000 mcg. in a liquid sublingual form(under the tongue as drops, spray, or dissolvable tablet). A diseased body could absorb the needed 1-2 mg. per day, which would solve the problem.

Doctors can diagnose possible Vitamin B-12 deficiencies with blood tests through reports on the complete blood cell counts (CBC) and the anemia panel, which measures the level of Vitamin B-12, folic acid and iron. The live blood morphology test can identify B-12 deficiencies. The red blood cells become shaped like an oval (ovalocytes) instead of being round and the white blood cells have fewer lobes than expected. Excess B-12 has not been reported as a toxic problem. Many vegetarians take Vitamin B-12 in a B complex twice or three times a week in a sublingual form under the tongue.

You do need at least four micrograms per day, which is a very small amount. Since your body can store Vitamin B-12 from five to ten years in the liver, we have an adequate storage capacity. However, excessive use of alcohol can deplete a years supply. B-12 is manufactured by certain bacterial algae (no animal or plant produces B-12). Some foods that provide Vitamin B-12 from bacteria would include one ounce of oysters that has five micrograms and two ounces of crab (5.7 micrograms). An occasional bit of oyster or crab sprinkled into your food would give you a source of B-12 . Two ounces of herring per day would give you five micrograms your minimum B-12 requirement for the day.

Supermarkets and health food stores now provide several grain products fortified with added Vitamin B-12. Nutrigrain cereal have fortified their rice and corn flakes, so one to two cups would meet all your B-12 requirements. Tempeh miso (fermented soybean) and tamari are both fermented by bacteria that manufacture sufficient B-12. Other non-animal sources of B-12 include the algae, spirulina and seaweed with bacteria clinging to its surface.

**Vitamin B12** RDA: 4 mcg. Supplement pills contain breakdown of B-12 and are not used as efficiently as the whole foods listed below. Friendly microorganisms (algae, bacteria) provide the ideal source of B-12 between 4 to 25 mcg./day. If the "intrinsic factor" enzyme (produced by your body) is absent, your body would not absorb this vitamin properly. The doctor may decide you need injections or sublingual form of B-12. Fortunately, this deficiency is rare. No toxicity has been reported by overdose.

| 1 cup or 2 oz. as noted | mcg. |
|---|---|
| Plankton - spirulina, Dried seaweeds | 160.00 to 100 |
| Oysters, Crab, Herring 2 oz. | 10.20 to 5.10 |
| Nutritional yeast, 2 tbls. | 4.00 |
| Nutri-Grain wheat/corn cereal B12 fortified | 3.00 |
| Flank steak, 2 oz., chicken broth | .68 to .24 |
| Miso (fermented soybean) | .17 |

## VITAMIN B-1

Vitamin B-1, thiamin, has been discovered to be very essential to good health. If you do not get enough B-1, it can lead to fatigue, loss of appetite, emotional problems, beriberi, excess hyperthyroidism, shingles and in severe cases - death. The RDA for Vitamin B-1 is set at 1 to 1.8 milligrams. It's important to take the B-1 as a complex, when you do use it as a supplement. A supplement range could be safe from two to one hundred milligrams per day. The higher dosage would be taken if you consume large amounts of alcohol or sugars. The lower dosage of two milligrams would be used as a preventive formula in combination with the other B complex vitamins.

To get proper B-1 from your foods, you could use sprouted sunflower seeds. Just one cup per day meets your entire Vitamin B-1 requirement. Millet, split peas, green peas, bulgar wheat, asparagus and brown rice are all good sources of B-1. B-1 deficiencies occur when people eat large amount of processed foods, such as white bread, white rice, sugars and alcohol. Because there is not enough Vitamin B-1 in processed white flour and sugar to metabolize all the carbohydrates. It's best to switch to whole natural foods, such as whole wheat bread with all its B Vitamins intact instead of white bread.

**Vitamin B1** RDA: 1 - 1.8 mg. Supplement must be taken as a B complex (with other B's) in range from 2 to 100 mg./day. The better your diet, the less you need supplements. The more processed white flours, sugar or alcohol you use, the higher the dosage of B's.

| cup or as noted (Vitamin B1) | mg. |
|---|---|
| Sprouted sunflower seeds | 2.84 |
| Millet, Split peas, Black beans, Green peas, Bulgar Wheat | 1.66 to .48 |
| Asparagus, Red kidney or pinto beans, Oatmeal, old fashioned | .24 to .19 |
| Sunflowerseeds (1/4 cup), Brown Rice, Mung bean sprouts | .18 to .14 |

## VITAMIN B-2 RIBOFLAVIN

Riboflavin is essential to good health, but it's the most common deficiency Americans develop. It is important for the maintenance of adequate antioxidant enzyme levels. The RDA has been set at 1.4 to 2 milligrams. To meet your needs, include the following foods that are good sources of B-2: wild rice, millet, mushrooms, collards, broccoli, various beans and peas. Deficiencies can occur, and they may show up as cracks in the corners of your mouth and children's growth also can be affected.

**Vitamin B2** RDA: 1.4 - 2 mg. B-2 is the most common American deficiency. Supplement range 2 to 100 mg./day.

| 1 cup | mg. |
|---|---|
| Wild rice, Millet, Mushrooms, Broccoli | 1.01 to .31 |
| Collards, Winter squash, Alfalfa sprouts | .29 to .21 |
| Split peas, Pinto or black beans, Pumpkin | .18 to .12 |
| Whole wheat bread (3 slices) | .06 |

## VITAMIN B-3

The RDA for niacin, Vitamin B-3, has been established between 15-20 milligrams. Niacin supplements raise the good cholesterol (HDL) and lower the total cholesterol. It can dilate blood vessels thus lower blood pressure while improving circulation. It has been shown help in the reduction of migraine headaches. 1 1/2 cups of broccoli would meet a majority of your requirements for the day. Sprouted sunflower seeds, split peas, mushrooms and beans are all good sources.

If you develop a deficiency of B-3 it can lead to pellagra, a condition in which the skin develops small spots that look like dirt or suntan. It can lead to paralysis and death. But, you can get too much niacin and excesses above 1,000 milligrams per day have been known to cause headache, liver damage and possible blindness. Time-released Niacinamide has been shown to be safer (between 20 -200 milligrams per day) however, don't exceed our recommended dosages. Any dose beyond this should be under the care and direction of a physician.

**Vitamin B3 Niacin** RDA: 15 - 20 mg. Niacin deficiency may cause depression, insomnia or pellagra (dermatitis, diarrhea, etc.). A safe supplement range is 20 to 200 mg. per day. Over 200 mg. of niacin may harm the delicate blood vessels in the eye due to excessive dilation. Niacinamide does not have this effect; but, dosages of 2,000 mg. may cause liver damage, depression and gout. Food is your best source, with supplements in moderation.

| **1 CUP or noted** | **mg.** |
|---|---|
| Broccoli Sprouted, sunflower seeds, Wholemeal flour | 9.7 to 8.3 |
| Split peas, Soybeans, Mushrooms | 7.0 to 5.7 |
| Beans, (pinto, black, etc.), Oats, Wholemeal bread | 4.2 to 1.8 |

## VITAMIN B-6

This vitamin is called pyridoxine and the RDA is set at two milligrams. It is needed to metabolize amino acids and for the formation of hemoglobin in red blood cells. If you eat two cups of brown rice per day, this would meet most of your B-6 requirements. Bananas are also a good source, as are chestnuts, one of the few nuts low in fat.

**Vitamin B6** RDA: 2 mg Suggested supplement range 2 to 25 mg. Deficiency symptoms are similar to niacin and riboflavin deficiencies - muscular weakness, depression, cracks around mouth and eyes, etc.

| **1 CUP** | **mg.** |
|---|---|
| Brown rice, Banana (1), Chestnuts | 1.00 to 5.3 |
| Carrot juice, Corn | .50 to .47 |

## FOLIC ACID

This is another important member of the B complex family. It is found mainly in green leafy vegetables. This vitamin is especially important before and during pregnancy. The RDA is set at 400 micrograms and if you take a folic acid supplement, we suggest you include it as part of a B complex. One of the best sources would be boysenberry. A cup would meet nearly one-fourth of your daily need.  Oranges, strawberries, tangerines, pears and rhubarb are other sources.

**Folic Acid**  RDA: 400 mcg. (.4 mg.)
Supplement in B complex up to 400 mcg.

| 1 cup (Folic Acid) | mcg. |
|---|---|
| Boysenberries, Corn, Cantaloupe, 1/2 melon | 83.60 to 45.50 |
| Orange, Avocado, ¼, Strawberries, Black beans | 39.70 to 24.70 |
| Tangerine, Pear, 1, Rhubarb..... | 17.10 to 8.70 |


## PANTOTHENIC ACID

Another of the B complex.  It is essential for the adrenal glands to produce their hormones.  In times of stress the adrenal glands can become depleted. Extra pantothenic acid  is needed to restore normal adrenal function.  If one is deficient in pantothenic acid is can lead to depression, fatigue and insomnia. the RDA is five to ten milligrams.  Good sources of pantothenic acid are mushrooms, brown rice, hot red chili peppers, cabbage, cauliflower and wheat bran.  Sunflower seeds when sprouted are another source.  If you take a supplement, a safe range would be five to thirty milligrams.

**Pantothenic Acid**  RDA: 5 to 10 mg.
Supplement range 5 to 30 mg.

| 1 cup | mg. |
|---|---|
| Hot red chili pepper, Brown rice, Sunflower seeds, sprouted.... | 2.60 to 2.00 |
| Cauliflower, Wheat bran Mushrooms .... | 1.60 to 1.54 |
| Cabbage, Chestnuts , Corn | 1.14 to 73 |
| Oatmeal, cooked | .50 |


## VITAMIN C

This is one of the most important and most remarkable nutrients.  It has a unique effect on the basic properties of molecules, tissues and cells.  It has a large range of metabolic functions.  It is essential for the production of collagen and offers protection from oxidative free radical damage.  Because of the collagen strength and the antioxidant activity, wrinkling and sagging of the skin is reduced.  Interferon production is enhanced with Vitamin C, which promotes immune function.  The RDA for this vitamin is 60 milligrams and you could get this amount from one orange. You might not be aware strawberries have twice the Vitamin C as oranges, broccoli has three times more, red peppers have four times as much and red, hot chili peppers have seven times as much more Vitamin C per cup quantity.

Remember, to get the most Vitamin C, it's always best to eat these foods as fresh as possible, either when they come from the tree or fresh from your sprouting jar. When you take a supplement, the range would be from 60-500 milligrams per day. In certain instances you may have been advised to take more than 1,000 milligrams by your physician, and if so, you should follow those guidelines.

Your body can store Vitamin C in your white blood cell buffycoat. Most people can saturate their storage capacity, if they get at least 100 milligrams of Vitamin C per day. A lack of Vitamin C usually only occurs if you're deprived of fruits and vegetables or in a more serious situation of starvation. This lack of Vitamin C can lead to scurvy - bleeding gums, sores, loose teeth, swollen legs and possible death. Take supplements derived from all fresh fruits and vegetables. This will supply you with a good source of Vitamin C and the necessary bioflavonid complex.

Vitamin C RDA: 60 mg.          Supplement range 50-500 mg.

| 1 cup | mg. |
|---|---|
| Hot red chili peppers, Guavas, 1 medium | 369 to 242 |
| Red sweet peppers, Black currants, Broccoli | 204 to140 |
| Turnip greens, Brussels sprouts, Kale | 139 to 125 |
| Green peppers Collards, Kiwi fruit | 102 to 89 |
| Strawberries, Cauliflower, Red cabbage | 85 to 78 |
| Orange, Asparagus | 50 to 45 |

## VITAMIN D

The RDA is established at 400 I.U.; a safe supplement range would be up to 400 I.U. It would be best not to exceed this amount, because too much Vitamin D could lead to a type of calcification of the arteries. In England this overdose side effect had been reported in infants. Now in that country, you can only get Vitamin D by prescription.

Your best source of Vitamin D is the sunlight. By stepping outdoors for 15 minutes, you will allow your body to produce all the Vitamin D it requires. It may be a cloudy day, but if part of your face and skin are exposed, you'll produce vitamin D. However, as we age, our ability to produce vitamin D in the skin declines, and our ability to absorb it is reduced. It is common for older people to have less exposure to the sun and poorer intestinal absorption. If liver or kidney or bowel disorders are present, you need a supplement of Vitamin D3 (cholecalciferol). This form works best with the parathyroid hormone to maintain normal blood levels of calcium. Vitamin D from milk is a less desirable synthetic form and it should not be depended upon for your health.

**Vitamin D** RDA: 400 I.U.
Supplement range under 400 I.U. 15 minutes outdoors in daylight allows your body to produce all the required Vitamin D. If climate or clothing does not permit this, a growing child would need a supplement or 3 oz. of fish per day (vitamin D is found in fish oil).

## COENZYME Q10

Coenzyme Q10 is essential for the production ATP (adenosine triphosphate) in the mitochondria. ATP is the molecule that our cells use to store energy. A fat soluble antioxidant nutrient, Coenzyme Q10 is not a vitamin. It declines with illness and with age. Tissue levels of CoQ10 are lower especially after the age of 40. Supplements of CoQ10 increase exercise tolerance and reduce angina. It can improve the strength of the heart muscle and reduce shortness of breath. There are reports of patients being able to avoid heart transplant surgery because of the dramatic improvements from taking CoQ10. It has been shown to reduce inflammation of the gum as well as stimulating normal immune function. Sugar metabolism in diabetes improves as well as the improvement of metabolic rate and the slowing of the aging process.

The amount of **coenzyme Q10** I take is 50 - 150 mg per day. In severe heart disease higher doses can be more beneficial. CoQ10 is not toxic although it is fat soluble. It does not accumulate excessively in the tissues.

## ZINC

Zinc supplements can help someone with vision problems caused from cirrhosis of the liver. It can also help men on kidney dialysis machines who have become sexually impotent. During the processing of foods much zinc is lost. Most of us do not obtain enough of this trace mineral . Colorado Medical Center Researchers have shown that if cereals were fortified with zinc much of the deficiencies from middle-income as well as low-income families would be eliminated. Good sources of this mineral are garbanzo beans, whole wheat flour, wheat bran, lentil and soybean sprouts. A supplement between 15-25 milligrams is a reasonable amount.

**Zinc** RDA: 15 to 25 mg.
Same for supplement range.

| 1 cup | mg. |
|---|---|
| Wheat bran, Garbanzos, Whole wheat flour | 5.60 to 2.90 |
| Soy sprouts, Lentil sprouts | 1.70 |

## SELENIUM

The amount of selenium in food varies depending on the concentration in soil where it was grown. The basic RDA is .05 to 2 milligrams. Onions, cabbage, carrots, potatoes, tomatoes, grains, cereals, fruits and vegetables are all sources of selenium. The Healthy Aging Plan is higher in selenium than most typical diets.

Some studies seem to suggest selenium reduces the risk of heart disease. Of course, people eating the most selenium were also eating more whole grains, fruits and vegetables, and as we already know, these foods are low in fat and cholesterol. As a result, it's not clear if selenium is the main factor in lowering the risk of heart disease. But, selenium is an anti-oxidant and can help improve and maintain good health by reducing the effects of processed foods.

**Selenium** RDA: 50 mcg./day (.05 to .20 mg./day)
Supplement range 50 to 100 mcg. per day (.05 to .10 mg.). Toxic at 5,000 mcg. (5 mg./day) long-term use. Foods vary greatly in concentration of selenium; depends on the amount present in the soil in which it was grown.

| SERVING | Lowest to highest in mcg. |
|---|---|
| Onion, raw (1/2 cup), | 1.3 (Maryland) to 1,513 (South Dakota) |
| Cabbage, 1/2 cup | 1.8 (Maryland) to 316 (South Dakota) |
| Carrot, raw, Potato (1) | 1.8 (Maryland) to 235 (South Dakota) |
| Tomatoes, 2 medium | 1.4 (Maryland) to 329 (South Dakota) |

Grains/cereals   Average 12.3 Fruits/Vegetables average .9 to 1.6

## IRON

There is more iron in the body than any of the other trace elements. The red blood cells, as part of the hemoglobin, are where it is mostly present. The RDA's for iron are 10 milligrams for men and 18 for women. The supplement amount also should stay in this range. Iron is needed to produce hemoglobin in the blood to carry oxygen and to prevent anemia, pallor and fatigue. Dairy products frequently cause iron-deficiency anemia by inhibiting iron absorption (American Journal of Clinical Nutrition 33:86, 1988). If this problem develops, stop drinking cow's milk.

Too much iron can cause toxic side effects. For example, an intake of over 200 milligrams per day has been known to lead to liver disorders. If you took in 3 to 20 grams per day it could lead to iron overload of the liver and possible death. The Bantu natives who do all their cooking in iron pots, have a tremendous iron toxicity problem because excess iron gets into their food. Iron overload kills more people, percentage-wise, in this culture than heart disease does in our country. If you are cooking with iron pots every day, I would suggest you alternate with other types of cookware.

**Iron** RDA: 10 mg. for male, 18 mg. for female. Supplement range 10 to 18 mg./day. Toxic side effects over 200 mg./day. Good sources of iron include sprouted sunflower seeds, garbanzo beans, lentils, parsley, split peas and seaweed.

| 1 cup | mg. |
|---|---|
| Hijiki, seaweed Wheat bran, Tomato paste | 29.00 to 9.20 |
| Sunflower seeds, sprouted, Garbanzo beans, Tofu | 7.70 to 5.70 |
| Soybean curd, Kidney beans, lentils, Parsley, split peas | 5.20 to 4.40 |

## CALCIUM

Calcium is essential to good bone integrity, to maintaining strong healthy teeth and for proper nerve and muscle functioning. The RDA has been established at 800 to 1,200 milligrams. This range can be easily met by eating a variety of foods, including turnip greens, collards, kale, cabbage, garbanzo beans, broccoli and corn tortillas. There is more calcium in five tortillas than in a cup of milk.

Milk is not a safe source of calcium because some people cannot tolerate the use of dairy products. Many races have an allergic reaction; the production of a certain enzyme is inhibited and the dairy products remain undigested. Some symptoms of this intolerance include diarrhea, confusion, and disorientation, bloating or distending of the stomach due to the milk or dairy products rotting in the stomach. I avoid all dairy products, including yogurt for over 25 years because I'm allergic, and I know I get better sources of calcium from vegetables.

You get more calcium, ounce per ounce, from vegetables and various beans and peas. Although the *Dairy Council* says you must drink milk every day and use dairy products regularly to get your RDA of calcium, this is not true. When you reduce your protein intake and increase the intake of complex carbohydrates, your body will absorb calcium much more efficiently.

Rich sources of calcium include corn tortillas, beans, broccoli and cabbage, etc. without the need for dairy products. When you take a supplement for calcium use an equal amount of magnesium. Recent studies by Dr. Anderson monitored people eating high fiber (with phytates) and found no effect (20 to 50 months) on mineral absorption. Levels of calcium, iron, zinc, etc., decrease slightly the first few weeks on the diet, and then stabilize as reported in *Diabetes Care (Vol. 3, No. 1 Jan.- Feb. 1980)*.

## A major killer in seniors - Hip fractures and osteoporosis

If you exceed 15% of your calories in protein, it leaves acid or waste product in the blood. As a result, minerals like calcium, magnesium and zinc are drawn right out of the bones to neutralize the excess acid, to maintain the pH of the blood. The penalty, though, is weakening of the bones, loss of teeth and an increased rate of fracture, which happens in our culture so frequently. Hip fractures have recently been considered the major cause of death in women past the age of 50. It has even surpassed the death rate from breast cancer. Once a person is debilitated from this fracture and bed-ridden, they may develop infections, pneumonia and other problems that lead to death. Osteoporosis is the loss of minerals from the bones, leaving them porous and susceptible to fracture and disability. One billion dollars a year is spent on hip fractures related to bone loss.

Women are eight times more likely to develop a severe case of osteoporosis than men are, and more women die each year from osteoporotic fractures than from breast cancer. Estrogen therapy can only slow the loss of bone for about eight years. Estrogen therapy does not cause replacement of lost bone. The use of progesterone cream is a much better, safer approach.

Exercise and a reduced protein diet are the most effective ways to reabsorb lost bone material. Recent studies reported women 50 to 80 years of age can increase their bone mass 2-3% per year. This can be done through brisk walking, light weight-lifting or other aerobic movements done at least 30 minutes, 3 to 4 times per week, In ten years you could reabsorb the 30% bone loss that usually disables women by age 75.

The Healthy Aging Diet reduces the protein of the average American diet from over 100 grams down to an ideal intake of between 45 and 80 grams per day. As you consume less protein, you will prevent acid waste products from protein-amino acid digestion. This is the key to stopping osteoporosis, because your body must maintain a pH balance of 7.2 to 7.4 or you would die. If the blood becomes too acidic (less than 7.2), your bones release calcium into the blood-stream to neutralize the acid. Calcium and other bone minerals like magnesium and zinc serve as a buffer. These minerals act as positive ions to offset the negative ions from acidic blood caused by excess dietary proteins (amino acids).

By consuming far less protein, there will be no acid build-up in the bloodstream. You will stop losing calcium, magnesium and zinc minerals out of the bones. In this way, the Healthy Aging Diet will prevent osteoporosis. This is wonderful news for people who want to avoid hip fractures, spinal column degeneration and loss of teeth, which is so common in the American culture.

The Eskimos of Alaska eat more meat and protein than most Americans. Their diet is 25% protein, the highest in the world. They experience up to 40% greater bone loss by the age of 40 than we do. The Eskimos surpass our calcium intake because they eat the bones of the fish they catch (over 2,000 mg. of calcium per day!) Yet, this concentrated intake of calcium is not enough to prevent osteoporosis. A negative mineral imbalance (more calcium loss out of the bones than is taken in) is caused by their excessive protein intake. Unfortunately, many Americans are mistakenly trying to eat more high protein foods like chicken, fish, nonfat milk, egg whites and animal based protein powders (found in weight loss drinks and body building formulas).

Ironically, if you use dairy products often to obtain calcium as you get older, you will be getting too much protein and probably will lose more calcium than usual. Other studies show elderly vegetarians who eat the proper amount of protein (40 to 90 grams per day) typically have stronger bones and teeth than meat eaters (as determined by X-rays).

**Simply reducing your protein intake and eating whole, natural foods can offset osteoporosis.** Dairy product consumers lose more calcium than they retain, according to *The American Journal of Clinical Nutrition (Volume 41, 1985)* women with osteoporosis were divided into two groups. Half were asked to drink three glasses of milk per day and the other half had none. After one year, the women drinking milk lost more calcium out of their bones than the women avoiding milk. Ironically, the National Dairy Council sponsored this study, and it showed the overconsumption of protein from milk offset the increase of 1,500 mg. of calcium in the milk.

The U.S. and Finland have the highest milk and protein intake in the world (90-100 g. per day) and the greatest number of hip fractures. Hong Kong and South Africa (black townships) have the lowest number of hip fractures - they consume the least milk and less than 80 grams of protein per day. Studies have shown if the protein intake is over 90 grams per day, the acid build-up in the blood will cause you to excrete more calcium through the urine than you can possibly take in, even if you take supplements. This loss of calcium and other minerals from the body is known as negative mineral imbalance.

Further studies of the Bantu natives in South Africa provide us with important information regarding calcium. The Bantu women give birth to an average of nine children and nurse each child an average of two years. You would assume these women need large amounts of calcium since they spend eighteen years lactating. But, their average diet contains only 350 milligrams of calcium a day. They eat mostly complex carbohydrates, whole grains, some vegetables and fruit, about a 10% protein diet. Because of this low-protein diet they have no calcium deficiencies, they have strong bones, they don't lose their teeth as they get older, their children grow up healthy and free of rickets and the other calcium deficiency problems that occur in other cultures. Osteoporosis, which occurs so frequently in our culture, is non-existent in the Bantu culture. How do they do it? Their diet is a well-balanced, nutritious combination of whole grains, fruits and vegetables, without the excess use of protein. The calcium they eat is absorbed properly and they maintain good health. Studies on people who eat grains, vegetables and fruit and avoid meat and dairy products have shown they have stronger bone density on x-ray than do meat-eaters.

Have your bone density checked for osteoporosis with a duel density photon scan. My bones are in great shape, even without using dairy products for 20 years! Read my books for the secret. How are your bones of the spine and hips? A simple scan is available at certain hospitals without a prescription, call us for suggestions.

We know osteoporosis can be conquered now simply by changing the diet and exercising regularly. We know exercise increases calcium absorption in the bones. To stop osteoporosis switch to the Healthy Aging Plan with added progest cream and quit smoking (just three cigarettes will draw calcium from the bones and start to deposit it into the arteries). Finally, if you're taking a supplement, stay in the 300-800 milligram range per day and it should be taken in a 1 to-1 balance with magnesium.

**CALCIUM** RDA: 800 to 1,400 mg. Supplement range 300 to 800 mg., to be taken in 1 to 1 balance with magnesium. Be sure to avoid excess protein, which depletes calcium.

| 1 cup | mg. |
|---|---|
| Sesame seeds, unhulled *, Seaweed, Corn tortillas, 5 | 1,740 to 310 |
| Nonfat milk, Turnip greens, Collards, Kale | 302 to 206 |
| Cabbage, Garbanzo beans, Pinto beans | 165 to 150 |
| Broccoli, Parsley, Oranges, Rhubarb, human milk | 120 to 85 |

- 1 tbsp. of sesame seeds has 93 mg. of calcium (more than 1 cup of human milk) and only 2.6 grams fat and 30 calories. Sesame seeds that have been hulled (outer seed coat removed) have lost 90% of the calcium.

**MAGNESIUM** RDA: 300 to 450 mg.
Magnesium helps to relax muscles after calcium stimulates muscle contraction. It helps to regulate body temperature, acid-base balance, absorption & use of other minerals. Small amounts of magnesium appear to help people with chronic insomnia, muscle cramps, headaches, depression and irregular heart rhythm. High blood cholesterol levels, high protein diets, diuretics or alcoholism creates an increased need for magnesium.

| Magnesium 1 cup or as noted | mg. |
|---|---|
| Millet, dry, Whole wheat flour, Beet greens | 369 to 106 |

| | |
|---|---|
| Swiss chard, Almonds (1/4 cup), Black eyed peas, cooked | 97 to 90 |
| Collards, Whole wheat rolls, 2, Potato, baked (1) | 84 to 75 |
| Yam, Oatmeal, cooked, Kohlrabi, Green peas, | 62 to 50 |
| Spinach, Prunes, Whole wheat bread (2 slices) | 44 to 36 |
| Banana (1), Corn tortilla (1), Cantaloupe (1/2), tomato | 33 to 21 |

## SODIUM

Sodium is naturally found in whole foods such as grains, beans, fruits and vegetables. Unless your physician has advised you to eat a very low sodium diet, the sodium level of these foods need not concern you. A diet composed of these foods, eaten in their natural state, will supply you with just the right amount of sodium needed for body function. What we are investigating here is the sodium level of processed foods - those jars and bottles, boxes and bags in your cupboard and refrigerator!

You may consider yourself already educated about sodium. You've thrown away the salt shaker and you only buy foods that list salt as the last ingredient. You've made a good start! But it's just not possible to guess the sodium level in a package by reading a simple list of ingredients. The only way to be certain of the sodium content is if the manufacturer has included a nutritional disclosure statement. Don't assume sodium is low just because it is listed last. Salt is concentrated, with 2,000 mg in one teaspoon. In proportion to other ingredients, it may be the smallest volume, yet still be much too high for your health. The United States government recently declared a standard for food manufacturers making nutritional claims. Foods advertised as "low sodium" may have no more than 135 mg sodium per serving. The manufacturer may claim "No Added Salt," but still use other compounds or ingredients already containing sodium.

## POTASSIUM

We need about 2,500 milligrams of potassium per day. The first thing many people say is, "I eat bananas." Of course, bananas are good sources of potassium, but did you know garbanzo beans are three times higher in potassium? Winter squash is also higher, and tomatoes are as high in potassium as bananas. Cantaloupes, carrots, avocados and potatoes are all good sources, too.

Potassium RDA: 2,500 mg. Fruits and vegetables are the best source.

| 1 cup or as noted | mg. |
|---|---|
| Split peas, Garbanzo beans, Lima beans | 1,790 to 1,162 |
| Winter squash, Tomato, 2 medium, Banana, 2 medium | 946 to 880 |
| Potato, 1 medium, Peach, 2 medium, Cantaloupe, 1/4 melon | 782 to 341 |
| Avocado, ¼ Carrot, 1, | 340 to 246 |

Whole natural, unprocessed foods have been listed that you and your family may currently be consuming fresh, or need to add as a source for nutrients. Certain foods (liver, egg yolks, cheese, etc.) were not listed because they are too high in such harmful substances as fat, cholesterol and salt. You would be smart to eat the other foods that are safe to eat.

## SUGGESTED SUPPLEMENTAL RANGE (per day)

This guide will serve as a summary to choose your supplements wisely. There are so many different products and name brands. I suggest you look at the vitamin and mineral labels dosages to see if your supplement falls into the proper range. If you find processed foods, extra sugar, white flour or alcohol slipping into your diet, be sure to use the higher end of the ranges for the B complex vitamins. It is best not to exceed the upper range by too much because toxic side effects can result. If you haven't used supplements before they may be used as a preventive measure. While the RDA's listed are a starting point, our safe ranges are based on medical research reports of deficiency from sub-optimal levels and on toxicity from overuse of supplements. Sublingual, spray, liposome, ionic, colliodial ranges are at the lowest end of the scale, because they are absorbed more efficiently.

**VITAMINS**

| Beta-Carotene A | 5,000 to 10,000 I.U. |
|---|---|
| B-12 | 4 to 24 mcg. |
| B-1 | 2 to 100 mcg. |
| B-2 | 2 to 100 mcg. |
| B-3 | 15 to 100 mcg. |
| B-6 | 2 to 25 mg. |
| Folic Acid | 100 to 400 mcg. |
| Pantothenic Acid | 5 to 30 mg. |
| C | 50 to 500 mg. |
| D | 50 to 400 I.U. |
| E | 10 to 400 I.U. |

**MINERALS**

| Calcium | 300 to 800 mg |
|---|---|
| Magnesium | 200 to 450 mg. |
| Iron | 10 to 18 mg. |
| Potassium | 800 to 2500 mg. |
| Selenium | 50 to 100 mcg. |
| Zinc | 15 to 25 mg. |

## FAT REQUIREMENTS

What about fat intake? You do need fat in the diet. **Linoleic acid** is considered an essential fatty acid. You only need about 2% of your total calories in linoleic acid, which is about two to four grams. You should not add oils or fats to your diet to get linoleic acid, because they are processed, and ironically, when you add oils to your diet it can deplete the linoleic acid and cause fat deficiency. Your best source of linoleic acid would be natural foods, such as whole sunflower sprouts and oatmeal. Two cups of oatmeal, two or three walnuts, five or six almonds or a tablespoon of sesame seeds are all good sources. Lettuce and small amounts of avocado are also great sources of linoleic acid.

Don't use processed oils to get your fat supply. To make corn or sunflower oils, for example, a solvent is first poured on the kernels or seeds. It is then heated to a very high temperature, and lye and bleaching agents are added. Odors are produced, so they add an antioxidant. As a result, a residual solvent is left in the oil, and then this is called "purified oil." Cold processed oil is no better; the only step they omit is the heating process.

You would not think of sugar as a good source of food. Yet sugar was processed from the whole sugar beet, and sugar beets are perfectly healthy for you. The same is true of corn oil; corn is healthy, but if you extract the oil, it's processed and loses its beneficial qualities. It takes 14 ears of corn to equal one tablespoon of oil.

If you must use oil in your diet, for cooking and recipes, rely on a very small amount of olive oil. It has a strong flavor and extends a long way, so you can use a much smaller amount. In cooking you can use non-stick pans or the microwave.

## FAT (LINOLEIC ACID)

Requirement: 1% of total calories; i.e.,: you need 2.22 grams of linoleic acid fat on a 2,000 calorie diet. Avoid oils and separate fats. Whole food is your best source of fat (see below). The best source of *Essential fatty acids* is derived from Flax seed, Evening Primrose, and black currant oil. One 500 to 1,000 mg capsule a day is sufficient to gain benefits.

| SERVING | Essential fatty acids | grams |
|---|---|---|
| Sunflower seeds, 1/4 cup, Walnuts, 1/4 oz., Oatmeal, 2 cups | | 2.90 to 2.00 |
| Sesame seeds, 1 tbsp., Avocado, ¼, Chicken breast, 1/2 | | 1.80 to 1.10 |

# VII

# Protein Myths

There are some myths surrounding protein. The most common myth is that egg proteins are a high quality nutritional source of protein. This has spread through the scientific community as well, and we'll help you dispel this myth. Do you still eat two or three eggs per week because you believe that egg proteins are a good source of nutrients? If so, you may develop several degenerative diseases later in life (if you haven't already developed them).

So why has this myth spread throughout our culture? Why do people believe eggs are good for us? Much of the fault lies with invalid rat studies.

In 1914 Osborne and Mendel did their first research studies attempting to determine which foods were the highest quality protein. They decided to use rats as subjects because rats have a short life cycle and are easy to monitor. They found when they gave rats animal-type proteins, such as eggs, meats, cheese, etc., they grew very large. In fact, when rats ate eggs they grew the largest. However, when the rats were fed potatoes, whole wheat, beans, peas or grain as their only food, the rats hardly grew at all.

Scientists thought there must be something nutritionally lacking in wheat, for example, because the essential amino acid, lysine, was too low in concentration to provide for proper growth in rats. *(Am. J. Clinical. Nutrition., 27:1231, 1974)*. In fact, when they added lysine to the wheat in a diet for rats, the rats grew suddenly. This began the idea of needing complementary proteins or complete proteins. You may have heard of people trying to eat beans and rice at the same meal to be sure they receive adequate protein.

Let's understand what this theory is based on. It is based on the belief eggs are of superior quality, because of the rat studies. But rats are carnivorous. They have sharp teeth and claws, and they have a short digestive tract designed to eat meat-type protein in and out before it rots. In contrast, humans have along, convoluting digestive tract designed to handle whole grains, fresh fruits and vegetables. Our teeth are mostly molars for chewing fiber.

Rats grow to full size in nine weeks time. Humans take nearly 20 years to reach full size. Rats need a concentrated source of protein (rat's breast milk is over 25% protein). In a follow-up study rats were given human breast milk and hardly grew at all because human breast milk is low (under 6%) in protein.

If a nutritionist were to analyze human breast milk based on this information, we would all be led to believe human breast milk is a very poor source of food for infants. Yet, as we all know, it's one of the best sources of food we could supply our infants. When children are growing at their most rapid growth rate, nearly doubling in size, human breast milk allows for maximum growth.

Let's make a comparison to food. Brown rice is merely 6% protein. If you give rice or wheat to rats, they don't grow very well. By comparison, we find children respond very differently. Children given various vegetable proteins, grow just as well, calorie for calorie, compared to animal proteins. (Knapp, *Am J. Clinical Nutrition. 26:586, 1971*).

One group of children at age *2-5* (a rapid growth rate period), were given only wheat proteins, which is *14 % protein*. This group was compared with children given egg-type proteins (which is a combination of wheat with lysine to make up for the limiting amino acids). The first group grew just as well, if not better, than the egg protein group. (Ready, *Am. J. Clinical Nutrition. 24:1246, 1971*).

The claim that animal protein is "superior" to vegetable protein is false. The truth is all natural foods of vegetable origin contain all the amino acids to satisfy human needs. The most recent findings suggest we do not have to combine beans with rice or other vegetables to get a complete protein. Frances Moore Lappe, author of *Diet for a Small Planet*, agrees in her 10th year revised edition that human needs are easily met without combining vegetable proteins. In 1988, the American Dietetic Association position paper emphasized it is not necessary to combine protein foods at each meal. The human body makes amino acids that combine in the intestines with amino acids from foods to meet our nutritional needs. Adequate amounts of amino acids and protein will be obtained from a high complex carbohydrate diet supplying a variety of grains, legumes, seeds, vegetables and fruit.

Researcher Dr. C. Lee reported a study (*Am. J. Clinical. Nutrition. 26:702, 1971*) in which a group of college-aged students were given two different types of diet, adding support to this contention. One group was given only cheap, starchy white rice, which consisted of just 6% protein. The other group was given chicken and rice. They compared how much nitrogen and protein was absorbed into the body and how much was excreted. Again, everyone was surprised to find the group eating the rice alone had absorbed 20% more nitrogen (or protein) than the group eating the chicken and rice!

There is something special about the vegetable proteins: they seem to have been designed more efficiently for our bodies. We absorb them better than animal-type protein foods. When Dr. Kempner at Duke University gave people protein intakes as low as 22 grams per day (a 94% complex carbohydrate diet from rice and fruit), the result was a protein-sparing effect. The carbohydrates eaten were used for energy, protecting the protein so it could be used for other essential use.

According to *Contemporary Nutrition (Volume 5, 1980)*, a group of men, weighing 154 lb. each, were given a protein-free diet, and the protein lost from the body was measured. They excreted about 24 grams of protein per day. So we know we need to replace at least 20 to 24 grams a day to meet a person's needs.

It's been established approximately 40 grams of protein would meet anyone's needs. If you make certain you get enough calories and carbohydrates it will surpass a person's requirements. Eating grains, beans, peas, fruits and vegetables provides over 60 grams of quality protein a day.

According to the **National Academy of Science** (1980), even a pregnant woman needs only 4 more grams of protein per day than a non-pregnant woman, which would be just 44 grams total. This would satisfy the total known needs of a 9 month fetus.

Another myth is that fish is a brain food. Although the brain does require essential nutrients, it's been found the primary source of food energy to the brain is glucose, which comes from complex carbohydrates. If you do not have enough glucose supplied to the brain you'd become very hypoglycemic. You might even black out because the brain is in need of the nutrients supplied by glucose. But, it's not really protein that gives us glucose, because protein does not convert nearly so readily into glucose as do the complex carbohydrates.

World-class athletes, including bodybuilders, have recently changed their views on protein. For years they have been telling us they needed large amounts of protein. Chris Dickerson, Mr. Olympia and winner of eleven other pro bodybuilding titles (he's won more bodybuilding titles than Arnold Schwarzenegger). Recently stated, "I used to follow a low-carbohydrate diet, which worked well enough for me to win Mr. USA, Mr. America and two Mr. Universe titles; but since I moved back to California in early 1979 to train for the pro shows; I've followed a low-fat diet since the body prefers to use carbohydrates for its energy needs. I feel more energy in my workouts when I'm on a low fat diet than when I was on a low carbohydrate regime."

Carbohydrates are your preferred source of energy. It's the high carbohydrate, low fat diet that is the best kind of diet even for a bodybuilder. Chris doesn't add extra protein foods to his diet. He has found he gets the protein from the whole wheat, beans, peas, fruits and vegetables in his diet.

Mr. Universe, Tom Platz, wrote in "*Muscle and Fitness*" (Oct. 1984), "If you're going to build an 'out of this world' physique, you need to experiment constantly. Therefore, I increased my consumption of complex carbohydrate foods and immediately noted an upsurge in my strength and size levels. My energy was increased and my blood sugar level seemed to stabilize. Today, I follow a high-carb, medium protein and low fat diet."

Natural Mr. Universe heavyweight bodybuilder Skip LaCour is

training for competition, using **The Healthy Aging Plan.** Skip is inspiring the world of bodybuilders to take drug-free training to the next level. Skip carries a Cool Tote so he can eat every one or two hours. He uses high quality supplements including DHEA, purified colloidal minerals and multivitamins. He also consumes raw sprouts, vegetables and fruits.

Mr. Olympia 1983, Samir Bannout, uses a high-carb (70%), moderate protein, low fat (10-20%) diet. So, many top bodybuilders are switching to a Healthy Aging-type plan. Tennis stars like Martina Navrotilova and Jimmy Connors also use a high complex carbohydrate, low fat, adequate protein diet. Dave Scott, who also follows this low fat approach, set the world record in the "Ironman" Triathalon (112-mile bicycle, 26-mile marathon, 2.4 mile swim). Carl Lewis, world's fastest man, near the end of his career switched to a high complex carbohydrate, low-fat low protein diet.

On a strict vegetarian or "vegan" diet (which includes no eggs or dairy products) there would be more than enough protein for muscle growth and maintenance, if an athlete ate enough foods to maintain his weight. I have followed a "vegan' diet, weight lifting, and running program since 1978. I get all the protein I need from raw sprouts, vegetables, fruit, tubers and grains.

Athletes perspire heavily and lose nitrogen in their sweat. While losing a smaller amount of nitrogen in their urine. Only during muscle building are small amounts of extra protein needed. This amounts to merely 25 grams (less than one oz) of protein, which is met by an increased intake of food to meet the caloric needs of the body

A gorilla is almost pure vegetarian! They eat tubers, grains, vegetables and fruits and they are one of the most powerful, muscular animals on earth. They don't need to eat meat to be strong.

In elementary nutrition textbooks across the country, there is a great misunderstanding about what our proteins needs are. In a textbook by Helen Guthrie, *Introductory Nutrition* there is a chapter about protein requirements. It has a picture of a big rat and a little rat and the caption reads, "For human requirements." The book states: "Rats will gain more weight on an egg diet than on a whole wheat diet" suggesting there is a correlation between weight gain in rats and tissue protein synthesis. If you read the chapter on protein there are no studies indicating what the protein absorption is when humans eat various foods. The only studies they support that give false credence to the assumption humans need eggs are rat studies! Why do they leave out the human studies?

We found out who sponsors the production of textbooks on nutrition: Huge budgets are provided by the *Dairy Council* and meat industry. They have found it is worthwhile to spend millions of dollars to teach our doctors and dietitians nutrition - based on those old rat studies! Further, they choose to include certain studies they want seen and leave out those they don't. It's a strong statement to make, but this has contributed to the worst epidemic of degenerative diseases seen in this country's history!

At universities, the *Dairy Council* promoting the benefits of eggs, milk and meat proteins provides pamphlets. We asked the professors why the *Dairy Council* is providing so much of this information. They responded by saying the literature is provided free and they can pass it out to their students so our future nutritionists, dietitians and doctors can learn "good nutrition."

What if you still decide you need more protein? Should you eat more chicken and fish and get as much protein as you can because you're getting older?

We have to disagree strongly with that idea. Our protein requirements are best met by whole natural foods. If you choose to add excess protein to your diet, the result will be devastating, starting with dehydration - a rapid loss of fluids.

Test this for yourself. It won't hurt you to eat a high protein diet for one day. Eat large amounts of chicken, fish, add some egg whites to your meal all day long. See what happens to you - you'll be very thirsty, very quickly. In a couple of hours you'll be surprised at the amount of water you'll need to drink. This happens because your body is building up excess waste products - urea, ammonia and uric acid from the protein that must be diluted by your vital tissue fluid. After several years on a high-protein diet you can develop severe gout, kidney stones, liver disorders and osteoporosis (a loss of minerals, calcium, magnesium and zinc from your bones).

X-rays of bones show us people who eat large amounts of meat, eggs, cheese and milk protein develop holes in their bones as they get older. By comparison, people who eat less protein and more complex carbohydrate foods have greater density and strength in their bones.

Now try another experiment. Two days later switch over to potatoes, fresh fruits, brown rice, whole wheat bread, spaghetti and other carbohydrate foods. Eat these for two days and watch how drastically your requirements for water are reduced! You'll also notice you'll start to feel better.

It is true we need protein for muscles, tissue repair, hormones, antibodies, enzymes and hemoglobin to transport oxygen and clotting ability. Protein is essential to life. Yet we get enough quality protein from whole natural foods that meet our caloric needs.

All vegetables contain protein. One cup of split peas or navy beans has 15 grams of protein, one cup of oatmeal or corn has over 5 grams of protein and two oranges have 2.5 grams of protein. Don't be misled by people who tell you these foods are a poor quality protein source.

You also may want to include small amounts of low fat animal products (and B-12 supplements) to your regular diet. You don't need animal protein, but some people enjoy the taste variety. These can be used as a condiment in stews, casseroles, etc. However, an excellent replacement for meat in any recipe would be "wheat meat" or "seitan." Wheat meat is available in some health food stores packaged in a jar.

Protein deficiencies (kwashiorkor) are due to starvation. A diet of whole, complex carbohydrates contains all the protein you'll ever need, as long as you get sufficient calories. Once you reach your ideal weight you will need to eat fewer fruits and vegetables and more grains, legumes, peas, nuts and seeds in sufficient quantities to maintain your weight.

**The Healthy Aging Plan** is a proven concept. Within several months you'll feel better than you ever have. This is an opportunity you will benefit from for the rest of your life. Start today.

**Protein** Requirement: 40 grams per day (up to a maximum of 74 grams). Eat enough calories to meet your ideal body weight, with complex carbohydrates to spare protein.

| SERVING | (Protein) | grams |
|---|---|---|
| Split peas, 1 cup, Navy beans, Black-eyed peas | | 16 to 13.40 |
| Flank steak, 2 oz., Halibut, 2 oz, Scallops | | 12 to 8.70 |
| Lentil sprouts, 1 cup, Collards, Brussels sprouts | | 8.40 to 6.50 |
| Soybean sprouts, 1 cup, Oatmeal, Green peas, | | 6.50 to 5.90 |
| Alfalfa sprouts, 1 cup, Kale, Shredded wheat, | | 5.10 to 5.00 |
| Brown rice, 1 cup, Yams, Asparagus, Cherries | | 4.90 to 1.74 |

**NOTE: Regarding sources of Protein**
1. Nuts contain protein and unprocessed fat with fiber that slows the absorption of fat, while providing a significant source of nutrients. Nuts are concentrated in calories and fat, so limit their intake. Raw nuts must be soaked over night to release protease and lipase enzymes. Seeds can be sprouted, which reduces their fat content to an ideal low-fat level.
2. Animal products should be eaten in amounts not exceeding (per day) 3 oz. of lean meat, 2 glasses of nonfat milk and 1 cup of nonfat yogurt. Reducing protein use will help to prevent dehydration, fatigue and loss of calcium, magnesium, zinc, etc. from your bones.
3. Eat a variety of whole grains (at least 2 different types per day), vegetables, fruits, beans, peas, nuts, seeds and sprouts.

**NUTRIENTS Needed per day for ideal health**

| Fat, Linoleic acid | 2 to 4 grams (1% of total calories) |
|---|---|
| Protein | 30 to 74 grams |
| Carbohydrate | 300 to 400 grams |

**STORING VITAMINS AND MINERALS**
   Don't worry if you can't eat all the foods I have suggested. By eating a variety and alternating the foods you eat from day to day, you won't have to worry about deficiencies because your body has a storage capacity. For example, your body can store **potassium** for one to two days, if you aren't getting any new source of potassium. You can store **calcium** from ten to twenty years, in the bones especially. Of course, you don't want to deplete your calcium, otherwise later, the penalty will be weakened bones. Understand, though you don't have to take in a calcium source every day. The foods we recommend have an ability to provide you with enough calcium.

This is supported by recent studies that show calcium is absorbed just as well by these foods as from other sources. **Iron** can be stored for four to five months. **Vitamin A** is stored from one to two years. **Vitamin B-12** is stored from ten to twenty and **Vitamin B-3** has a storage of two to three months.

**Sodium** can be stored about two to three days and the problem here is excessive sodium intake. Your body needs about one to two grams per day. We get all we need from whole natural foods. If you eat packaged foods that have sodium added, you'll probably add another one to two grams a day, but this is still a low-sodium diet. If you add salt to your food, you'll push it up to ten grams or more and then you will retain fluid and have other side effects. Also, you don't need to add sodium to your diet when you're exercising more. The body will adapt and adjust itself to conserve sodium as necessary, even if the temperature is very warm.

**Water** can be stored for about four days, and interestingly enough, has been recently shown to affect your endurance levels. It was found if athletes were deprived of water before exercising, they would fatigue much quicker. If they were allowed to drink extra water before and during the exercise, they lasted the longest. A third group of athletes, who could only drink water after they started when they were thirsty, lasted an intermediate amount of time. We have found now it's best to hydrate yourself before exercise. The rule of thumb is drink about a cup for every 15 minutes of intense exercise activity you anticipate and another cup for every 50 pounds of body weight. For example, if you weigh 150 pounds, drink three cups for body weight, and another two cups if you plan to exercise for thirty minutes. Those five cups may seem like a large amount, but you can function at your maximum intensity that day during exercise, especially if it's hot outside. Organic water from fruits and vegetables is best for ideal health. I blend up 64 oz. of sprouts and vegetables every morning or afternoon to get pure water, enzymes and energy.

**Carbohydrates** can only be stored for a few hours. This is important to know because if you don't eat frequent small meals, your blood sugar level may drop and then you have a hypoglycemic reaction. You'll be fatigued and tired, and then it's hard to get the glucose back to a good range. It's helpful to eat regular amounts of potatoes, grains, fruits and vegetables to maintain that glucose level. On our plan you may notice you'll eat more often because you have less fat in your diet. Fat sits in your stomach and has so many calories it takes away your appetite. Complex carbohydrates are burned efficiently and cleanly. Instead of eating three meals, you'll be eating four or five. It's okay to eat between meals and you should plan each day to do so if you want constant energy.

We store **protein** about six to seven weeks. We get a good source of protein with all the necessary amino acids from our whole natural foods. **Fat** is stored six to seven weeks. Some people tell me they store it longer than six or seven weeks and unfortunately a majority of Americans are obese and they wish they didn't store fat so effectively.

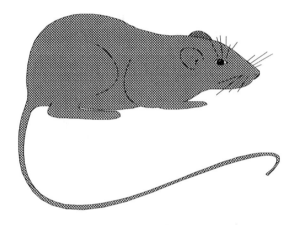

# VIII

# Enemies to Good Nutrition and Allergies

Some enemies to vitamin and mineral nutrition would be: white sugar, white rice, white flour, alcohol, cigarettes, antacids (they deplete various minerals) and baking soda (depletes the B vitamins). **ANEMIA** - It is important to identify the cause of your blood's reduced ability to carry oxygen first, and then find a solution that is best for you. Sometimes allergies to foods like dairy products can cause micro-bleeding in the intestines resulting in a severe case of iron deficiency. The red blood cells will look abnormally small shaped any carry less oxygen.

Unfortunately, in our society, processed foods slip into our diet, and we abuse addictive substances such as nicotine, caffeine and alcohol. This can deplete our bodies of B vitamins, which can lead to oval shaped or misshapen red blood cells. Cells that are small or irregular cannot transfer oxygen along the capillary lining properly. Because of this you will need some kind of supplement to restore the shape of the cells as new cells form every 120 days. We have found the Healthy Aging Plan of supplementation, nutrition and exercise can build up the deficient blood. Your need may include iron, B-12, folic acid, Vitamin E and Vitamin C, which can all be found in whole natural foods and supplements.

There are over 3,000 hidden chemical additives in foods. The average American consumes one pound of food additives per year! Monosodium glutamate, sugar substitutes, dyes, preservatives like nitrates, emulsifiers, fillers, waxes, tenderizers, texturizers, antiobiotics, and antifreezes are added to processed food.

Ice cream, for example, contains Diethyl Glucol, which is also used in anti-freeze and paint removers. A vanilla substitute, Piperonal, is also used to exterminate lice. A certain cherry flavoring (Alydehyde C 17) is used in rubber dyes and plastic; pineapple flavoring (Ethyl Acetate) is used to clean textiles and leather. There is a nut flavoring (Butradlehyde) used in rubber cement, a banana flavoring (Amyl Acetate) used in paint solvent - the list seems endless. Why don't they tell you these common food additives are solvents and are used in these products? It's because the food manufacturers aren't required by law to put the original name on the labels; they can simply say "banana flavoring" instead of its true name: Amyl Acetate. So, just because these names aren't labeled on your foods, it doesn't mean the foods are healthy for you. It's best to stick with whole, natural foods.

We also have to contend with the inevitable environmental pollution. In studies conducted by Cal-Tech, it was found we have a 500% increase of lead in our bodies, compared with prehistoric man. It only takes four times that level to reach a toxic level. We are at a borderline of extinction. That is why there has been a movement toward unleaded gasoline and getting lead out of paint bases and so forth. These heavy metals can build up in our bodies. According to the medical journal, Lancet, certain tests like hair analysis, can access the amount of toxic metals in the body. There are certain foods that can help remove these heavy metals. Foods high in soluble fibers, such as beans, peas, apples, pears, oat bran and corn flakes, seem to stick to heavy metals and reduce their content in the body. These foods also lower cholesterol, so you should use them as a preventive formula.

**Biomagnification** is the increased concentration of chemicals, pesticides and toxins that results when animals eat grains and vegetables exposed to pesticides, which concentrate 1,000 times in the animal's fat. When you eat the animal ' the pesticides and heavy metals like mercury or lead can concentrate in your body not just double, but 1,000 X 1,000 or one million times! The concentration of these potentially deadly chemicals increases the higher you eat on the food chain. Meat, fish and dairy products expose you to the highest concentration of these deadly chemicals. Grains, fruits and vegetables are comparatively safe.

Small fish and plankton consumed by larger fish like tuna or swordfish, and eventually eaten by humans, have potentially high concentrations of chemicals that are dose related. The higher the dosage, the more dangerous the chemicals become as they concentrate in your body to lethal levels that may induce cancer or liver failure. Meat, chicken and fish have 10 times more pesticides than plant foods: fruits, vegetables or grains.

Drinking the milk of animals (cow or goat) is equally dangerous because of the buildup of harmful substances that end up in the secretions (milk) of the animal. Dairy products (milk, cheese, sour cream and eggs) have 5-1/2 times more toxic pesticides than do plant foods. A woman who eats low or at the origin of the food chain (fruits, vegetables and grains) will be eating lower - fat foods with fewer chemicals, and in turn with fewer chemicals for her baby. According to the New England Journal of Medicine, March 26, 1981, only 2% of mothers' milk from women eating only grains, beans, fruits and vegetables (no meat) were found to contain significant levels of DDT and other toxic chemicals. By contrast, 100% of mothers eating meat and dairy products produced breast milk with significant levels of DDT, pesticides and toxic chemicals.

DDT poison was banned in the US, However, world- wide more DDT is being used today than at any time in the past. Years ago a chemical company spilled DDT in a lake in Florida. When the water was measured it was clean, however at the bottom of the lake the microorganisms were contaminated with DDT and the fish, frogs, and alligators lost the ability to reproduce lacking sufficient sperm counts. Humans now have 50% less sperm counts than was present just 30 years ago. How much more are we going to pollute our environment? We may not be able to control outside contamination, yet we can control what goes into our bodies via our mouth. And this is the biggest single source of risk when we consume other animals and dairy products.

Health-conscious people prefer to buy organic fruits and vegetables. Purchasing organic, seedless red and green grapes, potatoes, apples or carrots is worth the extra 10 to 60 cents a pound to avoid chemicals and pesticides. The average person eats at least 4 lb. of food a day, so for a mere $1.40 extra a day we will be supporting those farmers who care about future generations. This may force other farmers to begin farming pesticide free.

If you do buy non-organic fruits and vegetables, like cabbage or lettuce, then take a moment to peel the outer leaves. Rinse broccoli, cauliflower, nectarines, pears or grapes in water. You may want to soak them briefly with a dash of liquid soap or use one of the vegetable cleaner solutions currently available at health food stores. Peeling non-organic apples may be necessary, since the wax seals the pesticides onto the apples. It's far better to eat the fruits, vegetables and breads as they are, as compared to the fast foods and deadlier TV dinners. Less than 7% of the pesticides we consume come from grains, fruits and vegetables. However, 55 % of the pesticides come from meats and 33% come from dairy products.

**Supplements that will help with detoxification:**  Alfalfa, Bee Pollen, Garlic, Parsley, Capsicum, grape seed extract, Norwegian Kelp, Siberan Ginseng, Una de Gato, False unicorn, black cohosh, blue cohosh, cramp bark, pennyroyal, bayberry bark, ginger root, squaw vine, uva ursi, valerian root, blessed thistle, echinacea root, golden seal, burdock, dandelion, cayenne, chickweed leaf, slippery elmm, comfrey, yellow dock, mulllein and marshmallow root.

# Allergies

Allergens are the substances that cause allergic reactions. They can be caused by foods, beverages, chemicals and by particles in the air. Allergies may be caused by one of the following reasons.

We should be fed only mother's breast milk at birth and up until the first nine months of life. However, many mothers mistakenly think their baby isn't getting enough nutrients. Because of her love and concern for her baby, she begins introducing several foods from the table to her baby. You may have often heard mothers proudly commenting on how soon her baby could eat eggs, meat, cheese, or cereal.

This premature introduction of foods is nearly impossible for the baby's newly formed intestinal tract to digest properly. Large undigested protein, fat and carbohydrate molecules from these specific foods find their way into the baby's blood stream. The babies' immune system produces special proteins called antibodies to destroy the "invader" food particles and foreign bodies. By mistake, the baby's immune system may become conditioned to always react adversely to the consumption of those same foods later in life. We call these episodes "allergic reactions" to foods. This type of allergy problem may have been avoidable if infant formula or other unnatural foods were not introduced so early as a substitute for mothers' milk.

Mothers can cut their babies allergy problems by avoiding allergy-triggering foods while pregnant and breast-feeding. A study reported in *The Lancet* states that a mother may cut a babies' chances of developing allergies in half during the first year of life. By reducing contact with foods that are likely to cause allergies such as dairy products, secondhand tobacco smoke and dust mites, the allergy risk can be substantially lowered. Long term studies are needed to determine whether avoidance merely delays rather than prevents allergies.

In the study of 120 mothers and their babies, half the mothers ate no fish, milk, eggs or nuts during pregnancy. The mothers also avoided feeding their infants dairy, eggs, wheat or oranges during the first year. Instead, the babies received a hypoallergenic formula. This group also had their homes treated for dust mites. The other group took no precautions. After one year the researchers found the 40% of infants in families with no intervention had allergy problems as opposed to 13% of the prevention group. Infants in families with no intervention were more likely to have asthma or eczema. In both groups, infants who had one parent who smoked were four times more likely to have allergies - if two parents smoked, the incidence was almost five times higher.

Allergies also can develop because of genetics. In social regions of the world, people have become allergic to certain foods and their offspring will always be allergic to these foods or chemicals.

Allergies are not to be confused with an intolerance to certain foods, such as "lactose intolerance." A person may have a problem digesting the lactose sugar in milk. When a person has an intolerance to lactose they may have trouble digesting the complex lactose sugars. The undigested lactose sugars may rot in the stomach, sour and cause extreme gas, pain and discomfort in the digestive tract.

Allergies are different from intolerances because the food is actually attacked by your own immune system. For example, if you experience respiratory cold like symptoms, the white blood cells release powerful substances called enzymes and histamines to ward off or destroy the invader. These histamines will cause your nose to "run" and your eyes to "water" as a defense system. Normally, the invader would be a bacteria or virus and it would be expelled from your body or destroyed by your white blood cells and antibodies. In the case of allergies, your body makes a mistake, and gets set for battle against substances normally in the environment such as pollens, molds, foods or chemicals.

Sometimes a person may be allergic to a particular mold that routinely grows on certain foods. This person may not be allergic to the food, but after only 24 hours, the food; such as bread, fermented items such as wine, soy sauce or cheese may grow mold on it and cause a reaction.

To avoid mold type reactions you can store your food properly by immediately freezing those foods you don't finish eating at your last meal. Toasting bread helps kill the potentially offending mold. Also, purchasing smaller quantities of fresh foods, and eating them fresh, can help people who are found to be allergic to molds.

It is often very difficult to find out which foods you are allergic to because most food allergy reactions are the **delayed** type. A *delayed reaction* to a food or substance could show up hours or days later. The best way to find out what your allergic to is to find an accurate blood test which uses a persons own white blood cells. The **Prime Test®** for delayed food allergies reveals several different types of delayed allergic reactions, including IgG, immune complexes and white blood cell destruction. The Prime Test examines up to 220 foods and chemicals from a small blood sample. This test enables a doctor to help their patients improve their health by removing the underlying cause of their symptoms. Special slides with microscopic amounts of different foods and chemicals are examined under the microscope after a person's white blood cells are added to the slides. If the white blood cells break down and die, a food or chemical has been discovered that needs to be avoided. Sometimes you can avoid the food for a while to allow it to clear from your system, and then eat them occasionally to avoid a return of symptoms. Identifying delayed reactions to foods can help you to develop a personalized plan to free yourself of the stress and fatigue caused from allergies. For more information about this test, call us at 800-631-0232 or contact Mark Lovendale at Advanced health Center at 949-661-4001 or 888-Testwel. (His book is titled *Quality Longevity*).

**RAST allergy test** is another kind of blood test used to detect immediate reactions or acute allergies for IGE. It is best used for obvious reactions to molds, pollens, dust and food. Many other allergy tests such as **skin scratch** tests or *prick test* are less reliable or reproducible, and unable to detect delayed reactions. IgE acute reactions to foods generally don't need to be tested for by blood or skin test, because they show up clearly right after the food is eaten.

We suggest you focus on foods first, since you have a greater degree of control over foods than pollens or dust in the air. Also, by learning to avoid those foods that you are allergic to, it will reduce the load on your immune system. Now your immune system will only have to deal with environmental factors and with true invaders making it possible to fight serious diseases. Rotate those foods (especially grains) you can eat so your body does not develop sensitivity. Eat a variety of foods every week. Avoid eating the same food item every day.

This will strengthen your immune system. You will get sick much less often. In past occasions, when you thought you had the flu, you may have been actually having an allergic reaction to certain foods. This problem could have been lessened or avoided with proper understanding of foods that commonly cause adverse reactions.

You may be allergic to environmental factors beyond your control such as pollens, house dust or chemicals. Try eating foods free of allergy producing properties and you will be amazed at how much better you will feel. The elimination diet is a trial and error process described at the end of this chapter to help you feel better and to help you to identify any allergies.

If you are allergic to a certain food, rotating it, or eating the food on alternating weeks, will not stop your body from having a reaction to that particular food. Rotation diets only lessen the discomfort, because you are eating the offending food less often. To be cured, you must avoid the foods that produce an allergic. The following is a list of typical reactions caused by delayed food and chemical allergies.

**Behavioral:** irritability, fatigue, restlessness, hyperactivity, muscle pain, mental depression, bedwetting.

**Blood:** low white blood cell count, abnormal blood clotting, iron-deficiency anemia, low levels of serum proteins, low platelet count.

**Gastrointestinal:** canker sores in the mouth, stomach cramps, vomiting, colic, abdominal distention, bloody stools, intestinal obstruction, diarrhea, constipation, colitis, loss of appetite, growth retardation, painful defecation, irritation of tongue, lips and mouth.

**Respiratory:** chronic cough, middle ear trouble, sinusitis, asthma, tonsil and adenoid enlargement, runny nose, nasal stuffiness, hoarseness.

**Skin:** eczema, seborrhea, hives, hair loss, rashes, atopic dermatitis.

**Immune Complex Disease:** lupus erythematosus, rheumatoid arthritis, Henoch-Schonlein purpura, polymyositis, scleroderma vasculitis, periarteritis nodosa, milk-induced intestinal bleeding in infants, occult intestinal bleeding, gastroenteropathy, nephritic syndrome, pulmonary hemosiderosis, glomerulonephritis.

**Miscellaneous:** arrhythmia's of the heart, eye inflammation (conjunctivitis), generalized headaches, migraine headaches, arthritis, sudden infant death syndrome (SIDS, crib death).

Because dairy products contain more than twenty-five different proteins that are difficult to digest, they are the leading cause of allergic reactions. Most of the gastro-intestinal, respiratory, skin, behavioral and blood reactions listed above can be symptomatic of dairy related allergies. The incidence of **Crib death** is higher when mother or child is consuming dairy products. Dairy products have also been implicated in the development of a cancer of the immune system called Hodgkin's disease.

If you are experiencing headaches, hyperactivity or fatigue, it could be caused by dairy products or wheat. A low fat diet and slow aerobic exercise will usually solve most Americans' number-one complaint; fatigue. But, if you are still chronically tired after you reach your ideal weight, and you are exercising daily, then look for another cause such as food and chemical allergies. (Try this experiment - stay off all dairy products and or wheat for six weeks, then after this period, drink big glasses of nonfat milk and or consume wheat for several days and see how you feel). If you go back on dairy products and wheat, in time your symptom may comeback.

Colic is another problem caused by the allergic reaction to dairy products. When my son was a baby he was constantly crying. My former wife had already made a considerable change in her diet, non-fat milk, etc. I suggested she stop consuming dairy products altogether. She was not too happy with my suggestion, because she was breast feeding my son and not giving him any cows milk. She thought I was crazy! However, when the mother eats dairy products, the cows milk particles pass into her breast milk and into the baby's intestine and their blood. The cow's milk particles cause an allergic reaction that gives the baby stomach cramps, causing persistent fussing and crying. My wife agreed to see Dr. Fleiss, a top pediatrician and hear his advice. Dr. Fleiss is a professor at U.S.C medical school and is currently in private practice. He examined her and the child and told her to go off of all dairy products. The colic went away and our son was fine!

**Bedwetting** is another problem with children. In some children the allergy inflames the bladder, it enlarges and becomes insensitive to the feeling of fullness and this causes the frequent bedwetting. There are other causes of bedwetting associated with issues such as deep sleep patterns etc., however you can simply discover if the problem stems from allergies by having your child tested for delayed allergies or trying an elimination diet.

Dairy products are a leading cause of **iron deficiency**. Some people are so severely allergic to dairy products that when milk, yogurt, or cheese reach their intestinal tract, the intestines start bleeding without the person knowing it. It may change the color of the stool only slightly. There is a constant loss of blood, to the point where they become anemic. Many women have been taking iron pills all their life, but cannot stop the anemia problem. People go off dairy products, the blood loss in the intestine stops and they can then absorb enough iron from diet and or supplements to restore the health of the red blood cells.

**Asthma** is a severe breathing disorder that may be caused by acute and delayed allergic reactions. Many of our patients with allergies to dairy, eggs, wheat, etc., go off these foods and their breathing clears up. It doesn't work 100% of the time, but it makes such a difference that many patients improved to the point of being essentially normal.

A strange allergic reaction to foods can be muscle pain. Some people will develop muscle pain, others will get chronic pain from a type of arthritis known as **rheumatoid arthritis**. A case noted in the medical journal, *The Lancet*, was of a woman who had a thirteen-year history of rheumatoid arthritis. She was taken off all dairy products and within four months all the pain and stiffness went away from her joints completely. She then had one challenge test. The doctor fed her a small amount of milk and cheese and within 24 hours all the pain in her joints came back. It continued until she was off all the dairy products again. Many arthritics go off fat and the joints improve as the circulation improves, but many people under estimate the connection with allergies.

**Skin problems** including dermatitis, eczema and hives can be allergy related, as can canker sores. We have had many patients with skin type allergy reactions. They improve by avoiding such foods as milk, yogurt, eggs, shellfish, dried fruit, nuts, and certain food dyes. L-Lysine seems to help reduce canker sores because it helps offset the arginine. Arginine is an amino acids found in nuts and other foods.

The skin is an excretion organ that tries to remove toxic waste via the pores. The dead white blood cells form pus, acne and pimples to help remove waste out of the body. The immune system also may leave skin lesions as it battles allergens. Your skin may also improve dramatically as you reduce fats, oils, and sugars. As you identify what your allergic to, notice how quickly your skin becomes healthier.

**Vomiting** and **bloating** of the stomach are other problems connected with dairy products. When I was in my teens and early twenties, I suffered from bloating and **diarrhea** every day. I went to a doctor who prescribed Pepto-Bismol for my problems. Then I read that bloating and diarrhea could be related to dairy products. I went off all dairy products and within a week I began to feel much better, and after three weeks the bloating went away also. I no longer looked pregnant! When I bloated, my face and entire body got very puffy.

At one point I was drinking nonfat milk. Nonfat milk is much more concentrated in the milk proteins and the milk sugar than whole milk. I didn't realize I had an allergy to milk proteins and an intolerance to the lactose milk sugar until I did switch from whole milk to the nonfat. Even after I tried

"Lactate" to predigest the milk sugar, I still had a major problem with milk products.

I thought I was doing a great thing for myself by using nonfat dairy products. If you have an allergy to dairy products, when you switch from whole milk products to nonfat items, the allergic reaction may become more pronounced. Don't blame going to a lower fat diet, you are probably very sensitive to dairy products. When I was eating dairy products I also felt "senile," disoriented and unable to concentrate. After going off all dairy products I could think clearly and my memory was restored to a high functional level.

I remember one of our patients' who was about 70 years old. His wife had him on a low fat diet and one-day she brought him into our clinic. He could not even communicate and he looked "out of it." I reviewed his diet and noticed he was using nonfat dairy products. I suggested to his wife that they try eliminating all dairy products. In one month he came back in and I was happy to see the change in him and he was talking up a storm! His wife was very pleased with the results of this dietary change. His doctors had thought he was senile, but after the change in diet, he regained control of his faculties. I sometimes wonder about the diagnosis given to our elderly concerning senility. Don't underestimate the power of nutrition and what it can do for you.

Another major cause of **senility** stems from cholesterol plaques accumulating in the small capillaries and arteries in the brain. A zero cholesterol diet might prevent many cases of senility. Also, be careful to avoid aluminum from cooking pans, aluminum wrap and underarm spray. (Read labels - only a few brands are "free" of aluminum chlorhydrate.)

**Ulcerate of colitis**, a much more severe form of digestive disorder and **Crohns disease** also can be connected to allergies. If you are having reactions such as pain in the lower abdomen, gas, bloody stools, or constipation alternating with diarrhea, then try an elimination diet and see a doctor.

I have studied many cases of **infant crib death** reported in the medical journals that implicated the use of formulas that were dairy product based. Much of the evidence supported the hypothesis that an anaphylactic type of reaction occurred after the inhalation of the cow's milk protein. The milk was regurgitated from the stomach during sleep and caused the crib death. Babies frequently regurgitate small quantities of food during sleep and often leave traces on the pillow. This theory suggests that the inhalation of this material can induce a lethal reaction and that only a small amount in the lungs can cause death.

To support this hypothesis, an experiment was conducted on guinea pigs. The animals were lightly anaesthetized to simulate the sleeping child. Milk was taken from the stomach contents of cases of crib death and many animals died rapidly - they stopped breathing without any sign of struggle. The pathological findings in these animals resembled those of the babies who die of crib death.

In our country women are encouraged to use formula instead of breast feeding by the companies that produce the different formulas. This isn't too hard to do, since we live in such a fast paced society. In third world countries, however, the women usually breast-feed because they live a poverty-stricken existence and money for formula would be considered a luxury. But, in some of these poor countries, they started programs for the mothers to receive formula free for their babies. The babies would be weaned from the breast milk and start on formula. Many of these babies started dying suddenly from "no known cause." Also, many died of diarrhea related symptoms because dehydration would set in after suffering from diarrhea for so long.

Crib death is said to be of unknown cause, but I suspect we know the reason this occurs, not in all cases certainly, but in many.

Cancer of the immune system, **Hodgkin's disease** has been attributed to dairy related allergies. The continuous overstimulation of the immune system by dairy proteins may eventually lead to the breakdown of the immune system into this form of cancer. Consumption of large amounts of chicken has also been linked to this disease.

Many people try goat's milk because they have heard it is less allergy producing than cow's milk. This may be true for some people, however, milk from any animal (other than human breast milk), is likely to cause an allergic reaction. Try using lite- soy milk, rice milk or almond milk.

If you give up dairy products you can prevent **osteoporosis**. There was a study done, paid for by the Dairy Council, and after they got the results, I think they wished they hadn't done this study! Half their subject women were given two glasses of non-fat milk per day and they monitored their bone density by x-ray through the year. The other half was taken off all dairy products, no milk, yogurt, etc. The only source of calcium for the second group was corn tortillas, broccoli, beans, and so forth.

After the study, the group consuming the two glasses of milk per day had the worst amount of calcium and the bone density had weakened terribly! The group who consumed no dairy products had the strongest bone density and lost no calcium throughout the year. The study concluded the addition of non-fat milk and yogurt added extra protein to their system that left acid in the bloodstream and drew calcium out of the bones.

The body must maintain a pH balance of 7.2 to 7.4. If your blood becomes too acidic by eating meat and dairy products; you would die. The only way to neutralize it is for the body to release calcium and magnesium from your bones. The calcium and magnesium are positive ions to offset the negative acidic ions of the excess protein. So, ironically, the more milk you drink, the more calcium you lose through your urine. Instead of feeling bad about going off all dairy products, you can feel good knowing that your bones will be stronger and healthier.

Some studies show that fat in the diet is a major culprit in the development of **multiple sclerosis**, according to Roy Swank MD. Excess fats clump the red blood cells and restrict circulation and oxygen to the nerves. After 30 or 40 years of eating a high fat diet, it's no wonder multiple sclerosis is higher in the United States than most other countries in the world. In Norway, in those regions where a high fat diet is consumed, they have a significantly higher rate of multiple sclerosis.

By comparison, in the coastal regions, a lower fat diet is consumed, and though they are the same "genetic race," the incidence of multiple sclerosis is lower. The only difference is the fat in the diet. Dairy products are also suspected in damaging the myelin sheath of the nerves. It is believed that severe allergic reaction to dairy products or other foods may damage the nerves. Dairy products and fat should be reduced to help lower the incidence of this disease as well.

These diseases and allergic reactions from dairy products are compelling reasons to switch to non-dairy products such as lite soy milk, rice milk, or potato milk. Also, try the **allergy Elimination diet**, and just see and feel how much better life becomes for you.

For children, the elimination diet starts with brown rice cereal, rice milk, brown rice bread from the health food store (free of milk, wheat, gluten, eggs, soy, or artificial colors). Give your child a choice of yams, cooked non-citrus fruit like prunes, green and yellow vegetables. After one or two weeks if the bedwetting stops or other allergic reactions go away, then you know the problem is food related. Each three days you are to add a new food and monitor for any reactions. If all goes well, you can add it to the child's list of safe foods. Those foods that cause a reaction should be recorded in writing and put up on the refrigerator marked in red. The good foods should be put in your child's favorite color. Add to the good foods list from the Healthy Aging Six foods group of grains, green vegetables, yellow vegetables, potatoes and tubers, beans and peas, citrus and non-citrus fruit.

Here is an easy way to do your elimination diet. You eat the foods that are the least allergy producing for a week and allow your system to clear. If the symptoms that you were experiencing stop, you know it is probably food related allergies. You eat brown rice, non-citrus foods, yams, and a few other items we would list for you. After a week, you add in the first product you suspect is the offending agent - milk. If you get flu like symptoms, sore throat, cough, skin reactions, or emotional moody swings, you eliminate that food from your diet. You can then add wheat, do you get sick? If not, you probably are not allergic to wheat. You continue in this way adding in different foods to determine if you get a reaction. Some foods may cause an immediate reaction (IGE) within hours, other foods may cause a delayed reaction (IGG) one or two days later. Testing and careful analysis with an expert will help solve the problems associated with allergies.

Summary of the key points to follow while on the **elimination diet** to detect allergies:

1. Be sure to cook all foods thoroughly, because cooking changes the proteins in foods, making them less likely to cause allergic responses.

2. Temporarily stop using all condiments such as salad dressing, herbs, spices, mustard, vinegar, lemon juice, foods with artificial additives, colors, or dyes. You may use just a sprinkle of salt after cooking (avoid salt if you have high blood pressure, edema, kidney disease, or arthritis).

3. Under your doctor's guidance, stop the use of all medications.

4. For one week, eat only from the following foods. This will clear from intestines and bloodstream food allergens. These are the least allergic producing foods and substances:
Brown rice, puffed rice, rice flour, rice milk (plain), Brown rice bread (with no additives, no eggs, no dairy, no wheat), rice pasta.

Sweet potatoes, yams (cooked)
Winter squash (cooked)
Tapioca (you can make pudding if you cook it with rice milk).
Cooked non-citrus fruit such as peaches, prunes, plums, papaya, cherries, cranberries, apricots.

Green vegetables, cooked such as spinach, asparagus, string beans, celery, artichokes, beet greens, chard, lettuce.

Yellow, or orange vegetables (cooked) such as summer squash, beets, carrots.
Water only, no fruit juices, or soft drinks.

After one week of only the above foods, allergic-type reactions should be considerably less. If you don't notice any change you may not have food allergies. However, the only way to find out for sure is to introduce one test food into your diet at a time. Try adding each single food eaten in large quantities, several times a day, for two days. If you have allergic reactions to that food, list it as a food you can't eat. Wait four to seven days, by eating only those foods you are not allergic to, before introducing the next test food. You can test the fruit, vegies, and starches in the above list, by eating them raw, one at a time. You can build on the list of foods that are safe for you to eat after several weeks of testing.

Be sure to test corn, wheat, tomatoes, citrus fruit, strawberries, chocolate, and nuts because they are common causes of allergies of plant origin. The leading cause of allergies from animal based foods includes dairy products, eggs, shellfish, and fish.

Some people believe you can "rotate" the foods that cause an allergic reaction so you can gradually eat them again. This is not so. Once you are found to be allergic to specific foods by using the testing method described above, you will always be allergic to those foods. The solution is to eliminate totally the allergy producing food or substance from your diet or environment permanently. It will be worth the effort, since you will feel better and your immune system will be stronger, making you more resistant to disease and illness.

For peak performance and good mental health, avoid all dairy products and use rice milk, or soy milk. Avoid wheat products, barley, rye, and oats as much as possible and use the rice or the suggested grains listed above. Gluten is a protein in wheat, barley, rye, and oats and it is very difficult to digest for many people. This may be because the digestive enzymes cannot digest the gluten. The undigested gluten protein leaves an accumulation of toxic material in the intestines. This irritates the lining of the intestinal wall, causing constant indigestion and malabsorption of all nutrients. It is also possible that endorphins found in gluten compete with our body's endorphins (vital brain chemicals involved in mood).

Whatever the reason, weeks and months may be required before a marked improvement appears after wheat, rye, barley, oats, milk, cheese, and yogurt are removed from the diet. Reintroduction of these grains and dairy products into the diet usually produces a relapse in days, or even hours! This is why it is important to maintain a strict adherence to the diet and to be aware of the exact ingredients of many foods.

**Supplements to help with allergies:** Alfalfa, Bee Pollen, Fenu/Thyme, Lobelia extract, Melatonin, Una de Gato, Ephedra, white willow bark, golden seal, cayenne, peppermint leaf, Vitamin C, , grape seed extract, passion flower, wild yam, valerian root and L-Glutamine (2 grams – ½ tsp. daily).

# The Effects of our Diet on Earth's Resources

Are you aware that the majority of earth's resources are used for a meat and dairy based diet? Over 80% of all oats and corn grown are eaten by livestock and not by humans! The tropical rain forests are being cleared to allow these animals to graze. These forests provide an enormous source of oxygen to the environment and this destruction is causing a "greenhouse effect" over the planet. This in turn produces an increase in the earth's temperature and the atmosphere. This may change weather conditions, water and other vital nutrients that our planet needs.

It takes an acre of land to grow 30,000 pounds of potatoes, but that same acre can only produce 165 pounds of beef. Clearly, we can feed a great deal more of the human population if we started eating more potatoes, grains, corn, etc. It takes ten pounds of grain or soybeans for one pound of beef to be raised. Here is a shocking fact - it takes over 25,000 gallons of water to produce one pound of meat, but it takes only 25 gallons of water to produce one pound of wheat. Obviously, if we switched over to eating more sprouted grains, fruits, vegetables, and so on, our water consumption would be much lower and we would have more resources.

Our water is being polluted by many different sources, much of it from the dairy and meat industries, which uses 50% of our water supply. 33% of our raw materials, which includes fossil fuels such as oil and gasoline, are in short supply. It is estimated that at our current rate of consumption we only have about 40 years' supply left. However, if we shifted over to a complex carbohydrate diet, moved away from the meat and dairy products, we would have over 260 years of reserves left. This probably would give us enough time to develop other sources of energy extraction from the sun or other origin.

Pigs, cows and fowl produce 20 times the amount of excrement as the human population. All that waste by-product ends up in our rivers and our oceans causing severe mass pollution. 55% of our pesticide exposure comes from meat, 33% from dairy product and only 7% from plants. There is a great deal of publicity about grapes and apples sprayed with pesticides, but there is no discussion concerning the high concentration of pesticides in meat and dairy products. If more people were aware of these facts, they might change their diet.

As you can see, our choice of diet can dramatically affect our earth and its' resources. We need to educate our young people and re-educate our older population to the importance of these changes. We must return to a more natural diet for our own health and the future of our planet.

# IX

∞

# Strong Immune System Rejuvenation of Energies

---

We have been born with the most powerful defense system on earth. There is no single drug that has ever been developed that has the versatility and effectiveness that God has given us.

The principles that I described regarding recovery, adaptive energies, and your recuperative powers for muscle building play a major role in also enhancing the immune system.

At birth our mother supplies us with colostrum, a special breast secretion that passes on certain immunities to invading organisms. As a baby, you are exposed to friendly and or harmful bacteria, viruses, and chemicals from our environment.

Your body makes decisions about what is good, and what to fight against on an instantaneous and daily basis. This exposure to disease, allows our bodies the opportunity to become stronger with each exposure.

Our white blood cells decrease or increase in number and type according to each exposure. We produce certain special proteins, known as antibodies, to fight the same or similar future invaders. Our skin and digestive tract prevents passage of most of the unwelcome invaders and substances.

Our bodies have ways of dealing with bacteria, viruses, and chemicals that have gotten past our first line of defenses and into the bloodstream. We have bodily reactions to rid ourselves of these foreign substances. Symptoms such as fever, runny nose, mucus production, cough, sneezing, diarrhea, increase urination, pimples, and skin eruptions are good signs that our bodies are fighting to remove or kill the invaders.

A fever develops when our white blood cells fight invaders and release pyrogen proteins. The pyrogens act on the center of the brain that increases body temperature. The fever helps kill certain organisms such as influenza virus, measles, tonsillitis (infected tonsils causing sore throat). Fever also fights typhoid bacteria from contaminated water or food.

It is best to allow your body to increase in temperature to successfully fight the invader. Be sure to drink plenty of water to replace fluids lost from perspiration. Let the fever take it's full course. Wear light clothing, eat complex carbohydrates if you are hungry, consume fluids upon thirst, and the fever will do it's job.

Unfortunately, advertising and outdated myths have caused us to try to "break the fever" with aspirin, Tylenol, and cold baths. This fear may come from the belief that a high temperature will cause brain damage. In all medical literature the few reported cases of brain damage came from other causes, and not a result of the fever.

What you must guard against is dehydration. Excessive loss of body fluids during a high fever, could cause seizures or coma in the elderly. **A person with a fever must have a constant supply of water to prevent the dangers of dehydration.**

There are other causes of fever not related to infectious conditions. Dehydration, overactive thyroid, heart attack, or tumors of the lymphatic system can cause fever. You will need medical advice for a diagnosis.

Respiratory symptoms due to illness such as runny nose, sneezing and cough are ways in which your body expels unwanted organisms. The sale of "cold remedies" is an unfortunate lack of understanding of natural bodily processes. The attempt to control symptoms may potentially cause the illness to last longer! Be sure to use a vaporizer to provide sufficient moisture so that your cough is productive. Eat chilies, raw garlic, Tabasco sauce, salsa, and mustard to serve as a natural expectorant. You must support and trust your body and the inner powers that you have been born with to overcome illness.

I have known of some medical doctors who prescribe medications and tell the patient the drug will eradicate the illness in several days. When this comes to pass the patient thinks the doctor is a miracle worker. The drug and the doctor are given the credit. However, unbeknownst to the patient, the doctor knew that the normal course of the particular viral illness lasts exactly a few days. Several medical books, including "Merck's Manual" lists common illnesses, symptoms, tests needed, and the number of days the illness will last. This information comes from monitoring thousands of patients in past decades, with the same illness.

We have known for centuries about the incredible power of the immune system to fight disease and cure us within a prescribed amount of time. Your body's marvelous immune system should have been given the credit in most cases instead of the doctor or the drugs. The medicine cabinet is nothing more than a security blanket.

There is no known drug that fights viruses. Drugs do combat bacterial infections, but excessive use of antibiotics has created strains of resistant organisms. Your body can successfully fight bacteria and viruses without the use of medications.

In past centuries, sewage disposal was combined with drinking water. Contamination of water was a great source of illness and continues to be in underdeveloped countries. Starvation in third world countries also leads to a weakening of the immune system and susceptibility to disease. The recent decrease in certain diseases in our country is due to improvements in sanitation and public health procedures and not due to the use of antibiotics and other drugs, according to Dr. Denis Burkitt.

Infectious mononucleosis is a condition caused by the EBV virus (Epstein-Barr) or the cytomegalovirus. The mistaken use of the antibiotic ampicillin may worsen symptoms and cause a skin rash. Your bodies' immune system will provide for recovery within six weeks. The white blood cells known as lymphocytes become enlarged as the virus multiplies inside them. The symptoms of swollen lymph glands in the neck, sore throat, and high temperature go away as your body destroys the virus.

Many people experience chronic fatigue, depression, lack of energy, and feel sleepy during the day for as long as three months after recovery. This is why so many people have associated chronic fatigue syndrome with the Epstein-Barr virus. A blood test for the virus usually shows that the virus is not the cause of fatigue. We find that excess fat in the blood stream is usually the culprit in many people who complain of fatigue. Our low-fat diet and daily walking exercise will do wonders for the vast majority of people who suffer from fatigue.

Infants and children have an immature immune system. They will contract several illnesses during this stage of life. As your child reaches school age and contacts other children, the number of flu's, colds, and childhood illnesses will increase. You will find yourself getting many of these illnesses, as your children go to school. This is natural, however, there are ways to decrease the frequency and duration of illnesses as listed below.

Those people who have a high concentration of viral activity will find it essential to follow the guidelines of **restoring adaptive energies** to support the immune system such as:

1.  **Take several long slow walks** each day.
2.  **Sleep longer and awaken without an alarm clock** (go to bed earlier if you have to waken at a certain time). Avoid total bed-rest. It is important that you get up each day no matter how tired you feel.
3.  **Take several naps each day** as needed.
4.  **Reduce the frequency of sexual orgasm** to less than three a week. You can have sex with your partner, however stop stimulation short of orgasm. Preserve your sexual energy reserves to fight the illness.
5.  Meditate-avoid stress, avoid negative people & negative TV-news
6.  **Enjoy 80% water rich complex carbohydrate, low-fat foods.**
7.  **Avoid sugars, salt, or excess protein**
8.  **Avoid fruit juices, use only whole blended vegetable, fruit drink**
9.  **Nibble on frequent small meals** when ever your hungry.
10. Add **Homeopathic Human Growth Factors, DHEA, Testosterone** enhancing herbs, progesterone cream & Melatonin.
11. **Add herbs** including **raw garlic** to your foods. Garlic is an antiviral, anti-fungal, antibacterial agent. Add Golden Seal, Siberian Ginseng.
12. **Herbs, vitamins, ionic-trace-minerals,** Parsley, capsicum, Echinacea, Black Cohosh, Bee Pollen, Pau d' Archo, Red Clover, Norwegian kelp, Hawaiian Noni, Dong Quai, Una-de-Gato, Black Walnut, Ma-Huang, Kola-Nut, Cat's-Claw, Licorice Root, Valerian.

**13. Maintain a positive psychological state.** Think of a time when you were feeling really great. Now make that image larger, and brighter. How did it look, what did you see? Was something moving fast or slow? Think about what you were hearing. How loud is it? How fast is it? What was the temperature like? Was it warm or cool? What was your breathing like? Heavy or light? Was there an increase or decrease in pressure? Was there anything else that triggered a strong feeling? Asking yourself questions like this will get you into a more resourceful state.

If you keep falling back into depression you must take those tiring feelings and make them smaller and farther away. When you look at someone or something, make it look silly like a clown with a big red nose. If you hear something, speed up the tempo of what is being said. Make it sound fast by speaking like Mickey Mouse. If you feel something, change how it feels from rough to soft and smooth, etc. Change your physiology - sit-up, breath deep, smile, shoulders back, be excited.

By doing these steps, you can change the state you are in as it is stored in your brain from one of depression to one of high energy and better feelings. Keep asking yourself resourceful questions like, what do I need to do to increase my energy, strength and power?

**14. Avoid drugs: recreational, over-the-counter, and prescription drugs** (seek a second opinion from a **nutritionally oriented doctor).**

**Dr. Peter H. Duesberg** one of the worlds leading microbiologists from **University of California Berkeley** in his **book "Inventing the Aids Virus"** reports that virtually every case of death associated with AIDS / HIV is induced from drugs like Amyl Nitrites "poppers" used by homosexuals to have prolonged sex.. Also, drugs including Cocaine and Amphetamines cause the identical symptoms identified in people diagnosed with AIDS. Drugs are the cause of death. People that test positive for HIV and AIDS (the test has over a 40% false positive rate, meaning the people never had the disease, and the test was false!) are put on the deadly drug treatments AZT which will kill any healthy person. AZT was banned from chemotherapy because it killed too many people, rather than saving lives. Millions of dollars are being spent on research to discover the cure for AIDS, therefore, no one wants to admit the cause is self-induced and lifestyle related to drug abuse.

**Supplements that will help with the building of the immune system:** Ephedra, horehound, Echinacea Root, Zinc, Bee Pollen, Black Cohosh, CoQ10, DHEA, Dong Quai, Garlic, Parsley, Capsicum, Germanium, Hawaiian Noni, Hyssop extract, Melotonin, Morinda Citrifolia, Norwegian Kelp, pau d' Arco, Red Clover, Suma, Una de Gato, Vitamin B Complex, Vitamin E, Cedar berries, licorice root, uva ursi, golden seal, mullein, cayenne, grape seed extract, milk thistle, heperitin, narngin, rutin, quercetin, false unicorn, blue cohosh, cramp bark, pennyroyal, bayberry, ginger root, squaw vine, valerian root and blessed thistle.

# Rejuvenation of Energies

Your ability to rapidly recover after intense exercise (workout with weights, basketball, stair-climbing, cross-country running, etc.), a bout with an acute illness (flu, cold, etc.), an allergy attack (rhinitis, asthma, sinusitis), is dependent on your adaptive energies and your immune systems' ability to ward off illness.

Your adaptive energies can increase, by allowing for additional quality sleep, control of ones sexual energies, a superior diet, and stress to success conditioning.

Let's first discuss why sleep is so important, and what I mean by "quality sleep". Retiring earlier at night will provide you with more "quality" sleep. Wake up naturally in the morning without the use of an alarm. Darken the room you sleep in sufficiently, so the morning light doesn't wake you prematurely. Sound proof your rooms by asking your children, spouse, or other household members to remain quiet near your room, until you wake.

Taking an afternoon nap is a great way to add additional quality sleep, and the needed rest to do your best, and to build more muscle. Natural growth hormones are produced at higher levels when you are getting sufficient sleep.

Now let me explain what I mean when I say "control your sexual energies." Having sex, without orgasm, builds more energy. Your frequency of sexual sessions can remain the same or more during weight training and exercise. However, if you are having sex more than twice a day, then don't complete every love-making session with an orgasm.

A recent survey of over 4,000 males showed only a slight difference in the frequency of orgasms between different age groups:

## Orgasms per month

20 to 29 years old - 9 orgasms per mo.
30 to 39 years old - 10 orgasms per mo.
40 to 49 years old - 7 orgasms per mo.
50 to 59 years old - 5 orgasms per mo.

An orgasm more than twice a day, seems to draw on the body's nerve energy, and dramatically reduces our recuperative powers. Fortunately, 60 orgasms a month is above the study groups average. And it's unlikely that you'll have to worry about curbing your sexual appetite, if we recommend that you have less than three orgasms a day! Try having five to six orgasms a day and you will notice a reduction in your recuperative powers. As proof, your sleep requirements go up with frequent orgasms.

Your ability to overcome simple illnesses like colds and flu is affected by excessive orgasms as well. You will notice it takes longer to be free of symptoms.

Your immune system and muscle building depends on the same adaptive energies that are released after having an orgasm. So leave some energies please!

Thirty-four percent of the men on a high fat, high cholesterol diet, past the age of 65 become sexually impotent. They are unable to achieve an erection, and enjoy orgasm because the blood vessels in the penis are clogged with cholesterol. The cholesterol plaques restrict adequate blood flow to the male organ. This blood flow is essential for normal sexual relations into advanced ages.

In parts of Japan, when the farmers retire at the age of 65 or 70 years of age, it's very common for the men to take a bride of age 30 and begin a family. Their diet of rice, grains, vegetables, and fruit (with very little meat, and virtually no eggs or dairy products) allows the men to maintain healthy circulation free of any cholesterol plagues in their arteries. They also live long (age 90 to 100) enough to raise their children and see them graduate from college.

What a contrast from the typical American male senior citizen. He gets married at age 30, is unable to enjoy sex by age 55 and dies prematurely at age 70. The death rate from heart attacks and strokes is greater than 50% of our population due to high cholesterol, high fat diets.

Illness depletes our energy levels and our muscle building capabilities. This is because it takes so much energy to overcome the illness that your body will not have enough to build muscle during those times that you are ill. If you become ill with a cold or flu, reduce your training to simple walking. Long, slow walks will build up your immune system, and allow you to recover quicker from the illness. Also, walking everyday will reduce your bodyfat levels, and allow you to maintain your physique or figure.

Running or heavy weight training will be too large a draw on your reserve energies, and it will take longer for you to recover from the illness. Measurements of blood taken immediately after high intensity marathon running showed a significant depression in runners' immune systems killer T-Cells. People experienced a greater number of colds within a few days after running as compared to those who only walked the marathon distance. So temporarily stop training, just walk.

Also, total bed-rest should be avoided, if possible, because rapid atrophy of muscles happens within less than three days from total disuse. Our immune systems function at less than ideal, during total bed-rest.

Measurements of blood taken immediately after walking, shows the greatest build up of powerful killer-T cells and the immune system. This enhanced immune activity to fight bacteria, viruses, and cancer lasts for several hours after each walking session. Your state of mind will help turn stress to success, and enhance your immune system. Reduced stress, the way you view your life, and the positive thoughts you create will help you to reach your long term goals. The people you associate with will play a key role in your progress and fitness levels. Fun, loving, positive people, who share your common goals, rules, and beliefs help improve the quality of life. Remember, what you focus in on and your values are paramount. Other people are part of your life, they should not rule your happiness, only you can choose to be happy and vital.

You control your states. For example, sit-up or stand-up straight, shoulders back, breath deep, smile and be excited. Think of exciting thoughts. Say to yourself "I am strong, confident, happy, and vibrant." By exercising and eating properly, "I will feel great, powerful, and energetic." Your movements, posture, and thoughts can keep you in an appropriate state to workout, work at the office, or just be more fun for others to be around.

Your diet is essential for success in building a "hard body" free of fat. Your nutritional habits must center around high complex carbohydrates, less fat, less protein and less sugar. This will improve your recovery abilities. You will have more energy. You will require less sleep. High fat diets cause you to feel sleepy, and drain your body of vital oxygen. When less oxygen reaches the brain, you go into a state of semi-unconsciousness, and fall into a false sleep. We call it a false sleep, because it's not the type of sleep that helps build and restore your body. You may wake up several hours after eating a fatty meal and notice you still feel tired. Good nutritional habits will keep your bloodstream clean, fat free, and fully oxygenated. So when you do sleep, you will be fully rejuvenated and refreshed. You will need fewer hours of sleep to be fully restored. This will help to offset the additional sleep you will require during weight training, frequent daily exercise or challenges to your immune system.

The proper use of water is also very important to enhancing your adaptive energies. Many people make the mistake of drinking water all day long. Actually, the ideal time to consume lot's of fluids is just two minutes before you exercise. Drink about four to six glasses of water just before you workout or exercise. If you drink this much water too soon, you'll find yourself having to use the restroom continually. However, if you drink just before you workout, you find that most of the water will be absorbed into to your working muscles. This helps prevent fatigue and dehydration. Also, have water with you at the gym or out on the track, in case you get thirsty during the exercise session.

Avoid "sports replacement drinks" because they are high in sugar content. The sugar can cause dehydration, reducing your energy and performance. You can obtain the additional potassium and electrolytes your muscles need during exercise by consuming bananas, grapes, tomatoes, or potatoes as you workout.

Carry fresh food with you (try using a cool tote) so that you can snack more often. As you workout, you will need more glucose as your body is depleted of its glycogen stores. The Cool Tote is perfect for carrying a bottle of water, fresh fruits, and vegetables with you into the gym. I can nibble on fruit like grapes, nectarines, or vegetables like tomatoes to give me glucose energy if I start to feel weak, empty or hungry. Complex carbohydrates digest efficiently at the rate of **two calories per minute**. This replaces the glycogen stores of glucose in the muscles depleted by exercise. Simple sugar carbohydrates from fruit juice, sugar drinks, or candy, are absorbed too rapidly at the rate of **sixteen calories per minute**. Excess glucose from sugar can convert into fatty triglycerides in the bloodstream.

You may have been told not to eat before or during a workout, however, this is true only of heavy foods high in protein, fat, or sugar. Meats, cheeses, eggs, or oils are difficult to digest, and they leave a great deal of fat in the bloodstream. This will reduce the oxygen carrying capacity of the red blood cells and decrease performance.

**Magnetic Field Therapy-** is one of the oldest and also one of the newest ways to restore health and well being used around the world yet almost unknown in North America. Practitioners in ancient times in China, Egypt and India used naturally magnetic stones called 'lodestones'. Today, top golfers and pro football players sing the praises of magnets. The most popular magnets are the permanent magnets that are flexible and can be taped or strapped to the affected areas of pain or discomfort. Magnets work similar to acupuncture by opening up energy channels and increasing blood flow to affected areas. Although we don't know exactly how magnets or acupuncture works we do know magnets produces excellent results where other therapies have failed. Research studies show that magnetic fields accelerate the healing time of soft tissue and bones or joint injuries. Baylor College of Medicine showed 50 patients suffering from post polio pain, reported a 76% decrease in pain after only 45 minutes using ½ inch magnets. Russian doctors use magnets to speed up healing after surgery, to improve circulation and to mend bones. My colleague Julian Whitaker M.D., also recommends magnets. Sales of magnets world-wide are over one billion dollars. You will find yourself recovering more quickly after your workouts. In addition, your immune systems' ability to defend against illness will be greatly enhanced.

# X

# Feed Your Hunger
# The Easy Solution and the
# Cool Tote

Do you want to eat delicious foods (Italian, Mexican, Chinese and American), enjoy frequent meals without hunger, increase your energy and look fit for a lifetime? To have constant energy and achieve your ideal weight, eat low fat foods just before you get hungry.

Anticipation of hunger is one of the keys to the success of **The Healthy Aging Plan.** It is very important you learn to eat more frequently. We tell our patients to eat just before they get hungry. Be sensitive to that earlier signal of weakness your body sends you about thirty minutes before hunger. It could be a feeling of slight weakness, distraction or an empty feeling in the stomach. On other diets, you're told to fight the natural urge of hunger. Then, finally you're so hungry you lose control and give in to the greasy temptations of our fast paced environment.

Haven't you ever gone to the supermarket on an empty stomach and noticed how many fattening foods you bought? You know you should eat before going to the market. However, most dieters make a terrible mistake going to a restaurant or relatives house to eat when they're starved. Why not eat (fruits, vegetables or soups) before you go to a restaurant, a friends' or relatives' house for a meal? In this way you will be in control to avoid temptations and make better food choices.

Why do you think fast food restaurants are so successful? Have you noticed how liquor stores and markets have two thirds of the cash register area filled with candy and snacks? We have discovered your only protection from this powerful temptation, to control temptation, is simply to anticipate your hunger. You must eat low calorie, high fiber foods the moment you feel a slight drop in energy or have an empty feeling in the stomach. When you're trying to lose weight, you have to eat a lot more fruits (three to eight pieces a day) and a lot more vegetables - up to four pounds worth (raw, cooked, steamed, microwave or in soups). Vegetables and fruits are high in water content, so you won't have to drink eight glasses of water a day. Two to four glasses would be sufficient depending on how much you exercise. Many overweight people fear overeating. On **The Healthy Aging Plan,** a compulsive eater can "overeat" fruits, vegetables, soups and salads and still lose weight. For example, if you consumed four pounds of vegetables and fruit in a day, you would have taken in an average of only 550 calories. There would have been no room left for the fattening foods like meat, cheese, milk, eggs and oils.

An experiment was conducted requiring the participants to eat ten potatoes a day. They could eat anything else, as long as they ate the ten potatoes first (potatoes have only 69 calories each x 10 = 690 calories). The participants all lost fat weight during the three-month experiment. There was little room for any other food! Of course, **The Healthy Aging Plan** encourages you to eat a variety of natural foods, not just potatoes. The **Healthy Aging Plan** will work best if you don't smother your vegetables with fatty, oily dressings and cheese.

Veggies and fruits are so low in calories that they are actually digested within 15 to 45 minutes (the initial absorption of most of the glucose). This means the next meal should be every 15 to 30 minutes to get sufficient glucose and rarely longer than 90 minutes in between. You must learn to eat the moment you feel empty, weak, or slightly hungry. That is the signal from your body that your glucose level has begun to drop. The signal to eat will vary by how much and what kind of food you ate at your previous meal or snack. The constant presence of glucose will allow your body to bum fat consistently.

The Krebs cycle is a complex biochemical energy-producing process during which your body must have glucose to bum fat. Glucose is very important to the production of energy. If you don't eat complex carbohydrates to get the precise amount of glucose needed your body will actually break down amino acid (body protein from muscle and organs as a last resort) into glucose to get the necessary amount. Your body cannot convert fat into glucose quick enough to meet the body's needs. This is why foods high in complex carbohydrates are called "protein sparing foods". We spare the protein of the body by getting the glucose fuel we need from the food, allowing the protein to be used for its special purpose.

Complex carbohydrates should be eaten frequently to protect the body's stores of protein. Don't get the mistaken idea you need protein from meat and cheese when you feel weak (a common misconception). You are only in need of slightly more calories from complex carbohydrates with a greater food density, like grains. The lighter fruits and vegetables simply need to be eaten more often. Eating enough grains, breads, cereal and pastas will give you additional calories, strength and the necessary protein your body requires.

**The Healthy Aging Plan** allows our bodies to continue to use mostly glucose, along with a constant attack focused on fat in the blood and the storage of fat in the cells.

The quickest way to burn fat is to eat vegetables and fruits approximately every thirty minutes. The frequency between nibbles depends on how you feel, how much activity you're involved with and how big you are. For example, a big, muscular man who is also overweight and doing heavy labor, will need a higher volume of low fat foods than a small lady, who is slightly overweight, working at a desk. The big man will need more food in his stomach to feel good and get through his workday without undue weakness or fatigue. The smaller woman will feel good eating smaller, less frequent meals. It may not be practical to eat as often as every fifteen to thirty minutes during certain times of the day. If this is the case, then eat more bread, cereals, grains or beans that can sustain you for one to two hours before your next meal.

For example, before a seminar, athletic event or a prolonged business meeting I eat a bowl of cereal or two vegetable sandwiches, or one or two bean burritos (without cheese). After the two hours, I return to eating vegetables and fruit for the rest of the day.

Your comfort zone of eating also must be considered. There may be times when you notice it's hard to eat enough fruits and vegetables to feel satisfied. You may start to feel too hungry, weak or bothered by having to eat so often. At that point you should eat grains, breads, pastas, cereals or beans. This will reduce the number of meals you have to eat for convenience sake and will provide a feeling of strength and satisfaction.

Be sure the food you eat has a rich nutritional value. Make calories count! Your body needs fiber, vitamins, minerals, glucose, fat, protein and water. Which food do you think is going to supply these nutritional needs? Liquid diet drinks, which are loaded with sugar, fructose, dairy whey, synthetic chemicals and processed protein? Certainly weight loss is best accomplished eating nature's balanced food supply of fruits, vegetables, grains and legumes that are rich in vitamins, minerals and fiber.

We've become a desperate society bent on self-abuse and denial. People divert their attention from the need to eat properly by blaming the psychological aspects associated with overeating. Feelings of guilt arise from the resulting appearance of obesity caused by eating fatty foods. This vicious cycle of wanting to punish yourself through starvation for the "sin" of overeating can be broken by simply choosing to eat low fat, high fiber foods.

Follow the guidelines for **The Healthy Aging Program.** Forget the out-dated "four food groups" and starvation diets. Reward yourself, don't punish yourself. You will be surprised at how great tasting fruits, vegetables and grains can be and what a wonderful reward it will be for you to nibble each hour or two. All people enjoy eating and **The Healthy Aging Plan** will satisfy that powerful urge of hunger. The weight loss you experience will astonish you.

Large servings of potatoes, fruits, vegetables and soups are satisfying foods that fill your stomach's four-cup capacity. Compare this to very small servings of fatty foods that concentrate twice as many calories into your stomach. Your stomach sends signals to your brain when it's empty. Your stomach cannot tell the difference in calories; it can only report to the brain when it's empty. By eating frequent meals, eight or more snacks per day, you will not have as much of a desire for sweets or fatty foods. You will gradually recondition yourself into this new way of eating on **The Healthy Aging Plan** and become lean and fit for life.

The body panics when food isn't provided regularly and often "saves" calories by storing them as fat. Studies on food intake have shown you will lose weight more easily if you spread 1500 calories over eight or more meals per day, as compared to only three meals or less. Fewer calories are stored as fat when you nibble all day as compared to eating the same food consumed three times per day. Fasting, skipping meals or eating only one meal a day puts your body into a panic, increasing the output of certain hormones that encourage fat storage (adipocyte enzyme activity). You can control your body by eating when your stomach feels slightly empty, and you feel weak or hungry. Don't ever wait to eat until you're starved.

In the *Oct. 5, 1989, New England Journal of Medicine*, David Jenkins, MD, and associates proved the superiority of the Healthy Aging Way of frequent nibbling. People were given seventeen snacks a day, as compared to gorging on three meals per day on the same food. Several metabolic advantages were shown: The "frequent nibblers" experienced a significant reduction in cholesterol by as much as 10%, a 15% reduction in the "bad" LDL cholesterol, 30% less serum insulin output and 20% less output of C-peptide and cortisol in the urine. They also found the most effective diet in controlling lipids was the high carbohydrate, high fiber, low fat diet with 70% carbohydrate, 15% protein and 15% fat. In two weeks, The Healthy Aging type of program lowered cholesterol down to an average of 189 mg. People eating three meals a day from the four food groups averaged a level of 244. This fattening Weight Watchers type diet is 33% fat, 15% protein and lacking in sufficient vegetables, water rich sprouts or fruit with less than 52% complex carbohydrates served at the 3 meals.

**Supplements to use as an appetite suppressant:** Burdock, CoQ10, Norwegian Kelp, Stevia, Gymena Sylvestre, papaya, chromium AAC, Missouri snake (root), chickweek (leaf), licorice root, safflower, gotu kola leaf, guar gum, cascara sagrada, red clover, echinacea, fennel, black walnut, dandelion, hawthorn berries, L-Carnitine, yellow dock, psyllium husk, alfalfa, zinc amino acid chelate, Vitamin C, Vitamin B2, Vitamin B6, Vitamin B12, Garcinia cambogia, ma huang, panax ginseng,white willow bark, Ephedra and lecithin.

**Supplements to use as an appetite stimulant:**   Alfalfa, Bee Pollen, Cayenne, Gotu Kola, and Siberian Ginseng.

# The Cool Tote

Most people who are unable to maintain high energy or lose weight rely on fatty foods, without fiber. Great health begins with selecting high energy, low fat foods. This idea will save you money and time as you lose weight and improve your health in the process. Almost every person following **The Healthy Aging  Plan** who has tried this easy technique described in this chapter has reported fantastic results within weeks. Are you interested? Consider the following:

When you go to work or leave your home for more than a few hours, there is a tendency to eat whatever is available - candy, doughnuts, fast burgers and fries. As protection from fats and sugars, I would like to tell you about the Cool Tote.

Every busy person will benefit from this simple idea if used daily. Let me explain how this works. Get yourself an insulated bag with blue ice (Cool Tote) designed to carry food. Then, once every three days (twice a week) go to the biggest produce market in your area, and buy a selection of your favorite veggies fruits and breads. Take the Cool Tote with you wherever you go (especially to work and keep it under your desk). You can nibble on low fat foods when you feel weak, empty or hungry.

The Cool Tote idea allows and encourages frequent snacks between meals. Frequent eating from the Cool Tote to overcome hunger, overeating and bingeing may sound like a contradiction; however, it is actually an easy solution. In a recent poll, it was shown most people snack on extremely high fat foods (ice cream, potato chips, doughnuts, candy and sodas) between or after meals. Our approach - eating tasty, low fat foods all day long - will protect you from giving in to eating the wrong foods.

I have been training and educating busy people to follow a low fat, nutritional program since 1978. I found many ways to help people to comply with and follow the program, but none as effective or long lasting as the Cool Tote. For three years I helped thousands of people to follow the plan, while I only told a handful of people about my special Cool Tote idea.

It was in early 1979 that I hired Bea (Delgado) Campbell (my mother), as a health educator. She spent countless hours with me learning the ideas, teaching students and working with me to help participants follow the program. By the end of 1979, I hired several health educators. I noticed they always followed the program better than anyone else, because they were required to prepare the foods for our food demonstration classes for as many as forty to one hundred people. The educators had to make five-course meals complete with soups, salads, whole grain breads, main dish casseroles and desserts at least four times a week. They were encouraged to eat the unopened, unused leftovers. They followed the low fat diet perfectly because it was the only food they had in their refrigerator and kitchen. I also noticed the educators began carrying their foods with them in ice chests or sacks, as I had been doing for years, to guarantee the right food was eaten at all times.

The Cool Tote should contain your favorite types of fruits, vegetables and breads you enjoy eating. The average food sack filled with fruits and vegetables weighs about ten to fifteen pounds. If you want to lose weight, purchase those foods that are low in calories.

Buy vegetables that are easy to carry: a basket of cherry tomatoes, yellow or red bell peppers, etc. Eat the peppers raw and you will be surprised how refreshing and crisp they taste.

Red bell peppers are four times higher in Vitamin C than oranges, and green peppers are twice as high. White corn and yellow corn in the husk can be peeled and surprisingly, tastes mildly sweet when eaten raw. Take along one or two carrots and a small stalk of celery.

I also get vegetables in a jar like new potatoes (which are small, bite-size, and already cooked), green string beans and green peas. I take a spoon with me, pour off the juice and just eat the peas, potatoes or string beans right from the jar. Chinese snow peas are delicious eaten raw so take enough to last a few days.

You can microwave vegetables in the morning. Pour salsa, low-sodium

Worcestershire Sauce or mustard on them, take a fork in your tote and eat them on the way to work. Many of our participants put cooked potatoes - red rose or white - in a baggy to be eaten during the day from their Cool Tote. It's best to remove the skin from the potato. The green substance under the skin called solanine has been known to cause liver problems when consumed in excess. You can microwave your veggies at work if you prefer. However, many busy people have to eat on the go and save themselves time by taking a bite of potato or fruit at a stop light on the way to and from work.

You should purchase enough vegetables and fruit to last about three days. Some fruits take two to three days to ripen. Leave unripe fruit at home in a paper bag to ripen. When they are ready to eat, take them with you in your Cool Tote. A ready supply of fruit for your Cool Tote can help reduce the number of visits you need to make to the market.

Your Cool Tote would be complete if you make sure there is a variety of fresh fruit. Favorite selections for your tote can include Rainier cherries (yellow), or bing cherries, grapes, pears, plums, peaches and bananas. Bananas can be eaten daily on our weight loss plan because they have less than 2% fat and are relatively low in calories per volume. Eat fresh apples, nectarines, blueberries, blackberries and raspberries. Frozen berries can be placed in a lid tight container and eaten as they thaw during the day. The best way to design your Cool Tote contents would be to carry a variety of each fruit, and snack from whichever item your heart desires at the moment.

People who are accustomed to starvation diets, calorie restriction and skipping meals will be afraid to try this. However, you will find yourself several pounds lighter in six months without any deprivation, weakness or danger associated with those old ways of dieting.

**The Healthy Aging Plan** will work for compulsive eaters, busy people and all for whom diet plans have failed. Your food bill probably will drop dramatically, since you will reduce your expenditures on prepared foods. Also, you may find yourself routinely skipping restaurant stops. Most of my busy participants (Delgado seminar graduates and patients) go to restaurants for variety or for special occasions. As you reduce the frequent restaurant trips, you can save literally hundreds of dollars. On those occasions when you do go to a restaurant, be sure to nibble from your Cool Tote in the car on your way to the restaurant. By doing so, you will find yourself ordering less or no fatty foods from the menu.

If you're in the car for long periods or going to be in warm weather, you should invest in the Cool Tote, which is available in department or sporting good stores. The tote also comes with a blue ice packet to keep your fruits and veggies cold. You should freeze the ice packet every night and put it back in your tote every morning. If you travel and you don't have access to a refrigerator-freezer, just put ice in a plastic zip-lock bag with the blue ice. Place the bag upright in the tote and at the end of the day, drain the water and add new ice cubes. We cover the ice bag with one or two paper towels to absorb the small amount of moisture from the condensed water. At night when you get home from work, put the veggies and fruit into the refrigerator crisper. Leave them in the bag so you can just put them in your Cool Tote without delay. You must plan to carry your Cool Tote with you every day. Don't forget to assemble your foods in time for work the next day. The Cool Tote provides an easier, safer method of food transport.

It will be necessary to keep your Cool Tote with you, at your workstation. If you are unable to keep your tote near you, then take a banana, apple or some bread to nibble. If your food is left in the refrigerator, you may not get the chance to snack when your body signals hunger. Your busy work schedule may distract you and when you finally do eat, you'll be ravenous. You'll eat that doughnut, chocolate, cheese or potato chips that add fat. Just pinch yourself on your hips or waist! RIGHT?!

Nibble every 30 minutes to an hour if you're eating fruits and veggies to lose weight. When eating more grains, breads, beans and casserole dishes, you'll find you only need to eat every four hours. Remember sprouted grains and beans will sustain you longer since they are lower in water content than fruits and vegetables and are more concentrated in food substance. We encourage you to have a whole grain brown rice bread in your Cool Tote and eat at least two slices a day. You also need the high fiber, vitamins and minerals that grains provide for long-term good health. Eat from your Cool tote right up to the time you're going to eat at a restaurant or go home for lunch or dinner. You will be able to maintain control and select foods properly at these traditional set meal times. You may find you won't need to stop for lunch or dinner and many days you'll just eat straight from your tote. Consider the time it will save. Time that can be allocated for families walk, biking or swim. Take your Cool tote on outings to the park, beach or movies.

# Restaurants

When eating out, It's true some soups have more sodium than you would normally use (less than 200 mg of sodium per serving is ideal and not more than 500 mg is acceptable). However, the vegetable soups are usually so low in fat they make a great filling meal for faster weight loss. If the, soup is made with meat (chicken, pork or beef), you should spoon out as much of the meat as possible or when ordering, ask the waitress for less or no meat in your soup. Meat is dense in calories, fat and protein and is without any fiber, so it should only be used as flavoring in food and not as a main dish. Chicken and fish, also should be limited to less than a few ounces a week because they have as much cholesterol as red meat! Even if you remove the skin, cholesterol is permeated equally throughout the lean flesh of the chicken or fish.

I love to stop in for a tureen of vegetable soup at Marie Calender's. Sizzler's, the Soup Exchange and Soup Plantation also have good soups. At a Thai restaurant, I order Yum Won Sen (spicy salad) and Tom Yum Pak spicy lemon grass soup, which is my absolute favorite. I ask them to substitute broccoli for the large amount of chicken they traditionally use. At Mexican restaurants, I order tortilla soup without cheese or chicken, albondigas soup without meatballs, black bean soup without sour cream or gazpacho soup (a cold traditional Spanish soup made with tomatoes, onions and vegetables).

**VEGETABLES:** All vegetables are fine when served without butter, margarine or oil. Try a steamed artichoke or a baked potato -with meatless tomato sauce.

**Fruit:** A fruit salad or fresh fruit is good for dessert

## CHINESE, JAPANESE OR THAI
When you order, request no oil, eggs, M. S.G., sugar, or soy sauce.

**VEGETABLES:** Ask them to stir fry, your vegetables in chicken or fish stock They can, add cornstarch to thicken and ginger and garlic to flavor. Hot mustard is good to use at the table. Try to select soups and vegetables with broccoli added instead of meat. However, you can have approximately 3 oz. of chicken or fish with your vegetables two or -three times per week. Avoid beef, pork and duck. Order chop suey or chow mein with very little oil. For taste variety, try the spicy hot Szechwan sauces on broccoli, eggplant or other vegetables.

**RICE:** Choose plain steamed rice instead of fried rice. It is browned by frying in soy sauce or oil. Avoid hors d'oeuvres because they are high in fat and cholesterol.

## MEXICAN

Call ahead in the morning to order beans without lard; they may oblige you.

**SOUP:** Gazpacho, a cold vegetable soup, is good to start the meal. Also, Albondigas soup without meatballs or tortilla soup without the cheese.

**SALAD:** Try a dinner salad with. fresh lemon and salsa.

**CORN TORTILLAS:** Request, 1/2 dozen soft and steamed to dip in the salsa. Avoid fried chips. (If they are crispy, they are fried).

**ENTREE:** Try enchiladas stuffed with rice and no cheese. Try a tostada - ask for a steamed corn tortilla bottom instead of fried. Top with plain beans, shredded lettuce, onion, salsa and just a dab of guacamole.

**FAJITA VEGETABLES:** Stir fried without oil, beans cooked in water, corn tortillas.

**BURRITOS:** Without cheese, add hot sauce to taste

## FRENCH

**APPETIZERS:** Vegetables in a light vinaigrette, vegetable relish, French bread.

**SALADS:** Salads of fresh or steamed vegetables, Salad Nicoise without oil or egg yolk may be a safe choice.

**ENTREE:** Ratatouille (cooked vegetables), a simple vegetable soufflé made with egg whites (without the butter), or a baked potato with chives are all tasty choices. Most restaurants will prepare a beautiful steamed vegetable plate to order even if it is not on the menu. Request no salt, butter, margarine, oil or sauces. If your cholesterol level is below 160, you may order broiled fish chicken (or frog legs) once or twice a week.

## AMERICAN

**SALAD/SALAD BARS:** Fresh vegetables are unlimited. Limit the marinated vegetables, as they may be salted. Request tasty vegetable soups, also try fruit salads. Avoid eggs, meat, excess chicken, turkey, cheese, oil or mayonnaise based salad dressings, and bacon bits. Try using lemon juice with garlic and herbs, if available.

**BREAD:** Try for sprouted whole grain bread or rolls, but if they are not available, anything other than butter or egg bread will do.

**ENTREE:** Steamed vegetable plate can usually be ordered, even if it is not on the menu. Ask them to omit the butter, oil, margarine and sauces. A side order of baked potato (request chili salsa instead of butter) or the fresh vegetables of the day can be an excellent main course after the salad bar. You'll leave feeling full, knowing you haven't over stressed your body.

**DESSERT:** Try fresh fruit or fruit salad. Fruit sorbet is good, too. If you feel very decadent, split a rich dessert among several people - and take tiny bites.

## BREAKFAST BONUSES:

- Ask for sugar and salt-free cereals such as Rice crispies, oatmeal, Cream of Wheat, or Grape-Nuts.
- Try apple juice with water added instead of nonfat milk on cereal!
- Fresh fruit can generally be found at most coffee shops or breakfast houses. Order 1/2 grapefruit, orange sections, melon in season or sliced bananas.
- Always ask for dry toast or rolls, since most restaurants butter your toast for you. If you must, use jam for a spread on toast instead of butter.

## LUNCH TIME SAVERS:

- Have hot soup, broth based instead of creamed, as a main part of you lunch Always order sandwiches on whole grain bread and  hold the mayo.

Look for eating places that offer minimally processed foods. Cafeterias - and lunch counters have the advantage of showing you exactly what you are getting. The trick is to choose foods that are not swimming in fat, oil or sugar. Natural and vegetarian restaurants are good choices. They offer fresh vegetables and fruit salads, fruit and vegetable juices, whole grain breads, vegetable casseroles, etc. Beware of dishes laden with cheese, eggs or oil.

- Try creating your own vegetable sandwich with pita bread or crusty rolls, filled with lettuce, tomatoes, pickles, beans, nice, pasta, cucumbers, carrots, or cauliflower.
- Pick a fast food restaurant with a salad bar so you can, fill up on, raw vegetables. Otherwise order the simplest sandwich;  leave off the fat-rich hamburger or chicken meat, instead request the bun, lettuce, tomatoes, pickles, mustard, catsup and hold the mayo; eat french fries on a limited basis (surprisingly  fries may have less total fat than cheeseburgers or cheese tacos); order fruit juice instead of a milkshake (fast food restaurants probably will not have nonfat milk).
- Mashed potatoes (hold the gravy) with several ears of corn (hold the butter) can be a filling and healthy alternative to chicken.

## RESTAURANT DINNER, PREPARATIONS:
- Call the restaurant in advance for special requests. This courtesy will improve your chances, of getting what you want. The worst that can happen is the restaurant will refuse. In that case, pick another restaurant.
- Eat something before you leave home and nibble from your Cool Tote in route to the restaurant, It will take the edge off your appetite so that fat laden temptations will not be as difficult to refuse.
- Think before entering. Have a good idea what you will order before you enter a restaurant- then stick to it. Try new dishes only if they fit your basic plan.
- Order a la carte to avoid unwanted courses and trimmings.
- Think in terms of low fat versus high fat choices for each course. For example, if appetizers are placed on the table, concentrate on celery and carrots instead of cheese, or for soup, choose hot consommé over cold vichyssoise
- Order meatless dishes. Emphasize vegetables. Choose broiled or baked foods - not fried or french fried.
- Don't be afraid to split a meal with a friend.
- Skip dessert or have fresh fruit in season.

155

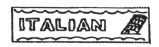

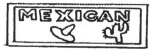

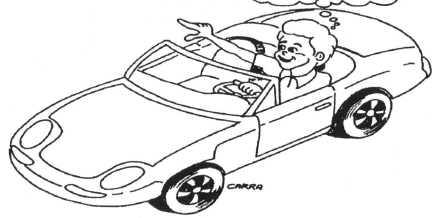

# XI

∞

# Rules for Fast Fat Loss

---

In the United States today, obesity effects more than 70 million Americans, and taken as a whole, we carry around 2.3 billion pounds excess body fat! To achieve Optimum Weight Control, we must choose a water rich high carbohydrate, low fat, high-fiber diet combined with a consistent exercise program. Let's first discuss our diet as compared to those of other countries.

In our country, only 22% of our diet is composed of complex carbohydrates (unprocessed whole grains, beans, fruits and vegetables) and as a result, over 32% of our people are obese. In countries such as Uruguay and Venezuela where they eat a diet higher (53-60%) in fiber and starchy complex carbohydrates, only 20% of the people are overweight. Yet when you examine countries where the diet is composed of over 70-80% complex carbohydrates, obesity is almost nonexistent.

**THE FIRST RULE** for weight loss is simple: The more water rich complex carbohydrates (potatoes, fruits, vegetables, salads, spaghetti squash, etc.) you eat, the more likely you'll have an ideal body weight.

**THE SECOND RULE** is to eat large amounts of soups because they are filling and satisfying. Make very thick, flavorful vegetable soups and you will lose fat weight quickly, without being hungry.

**THE THIRD RULE** would be to keep several containers of chopped vegetables in your refrigerator. These vegetables can be used to make large salads and casseroles. When you begin using a large serving bowl in place of a small, standard size bowl, you will be eating your way to a more slender body!

**THE FOURTH RULE is to eat** more fruit, because fruit (like vegetables) is high in water content and high in fiber, both of which have almost no calories. Even watermelon is a good weight loss food (along with apples, pears, nectarines, oranges, etc.) You will lose fat if you snack on fruit and vegetables constantly, day and night, with meals or between meals. If you have a sweet tooth and you have trouble resisting fatty candy bars, try consuming fruit like cherries, blueberries, grapes and watermelon in place of those sweets. You will still get those cravings for candy; however, if you have a ready supply of fruit to eat at all times, then you can successfully resist temptations.

**THE FIFTH RULE** of weight control is by **reducing fat** you reduce calories. Every gram of fat has 9 calories. Yet every gram of carbohydrate or protein provides just 4 calories. Remember, fats have 2 1/4 times more calories which is why they're called "fats" and why they are so "fattening". Read labels on the foods you buy to be sure you're eating less than 45 grams of fat per day. On a 2,000-calorie diet this works out to be 20% fat; on a 1,000-calorie weight loss diet, you should eat less than 22 grams of fat daily. Generally, a food should contain less than four grams of fat per one-cup serving. You must limit or avoid fats, oils, margarine, eggs, low fat and whole milk, cheese, peanut butter and fatty meats.

**THE SIXTH RULE** to weight control is to be sure to eat more foods **high in fiber** and low in food density. Your stomach can hold about four cups of food before a signal is sent to the brain that tells you that you're full. If you begin eating large amounts of complex carbohydrates that are naturally high in fiber, most of the food you eat will be **low in food density** and very low in calories. This is because fiber by definition is non-digestible. Because you can't digest fiber for calories, it just passes out of the body. For example, your stomach capacity would be fully satisfied throughout the day if you ate four cups of food for breakfast (blended vegetable and fruit drink), four cups of food for lunch (salad bar of vegetables and fruit, sandwich of sprouted whole grain bread with veggies or beans inside), and four cups of dinner (salad bar, soup, fruit, potato, corn and Spanish brown rice). You may add light snacks of veggies and fruit between meals. The best thing is even with all this tasty food you would have only consumed about 900 to 1600 calories for the day! This would allow you to lose weight at a safe and healthful pace, free of hunger.

158

Always ask yourself these questions: Does this food contain fiber? Is it of plant origin? Is it unprocessed? For example, do cheese, steak, chicken, fish, milk, yogurt, eggs, hamburgers, mayonnaise or vegetable oil have fiber in them? The answer is no. Foods of animal origin have no fiber. They are totally digested and absorbed as calories. Foods like sugar and vegetable oil have lost their fiber through man-made processing. One of the worst examples of man's intervention into Mother Nature's food supply is corn oil. It takes over 14 ears of corn to make one tablespoon of oil! These concentrated foods are fattening because Westerners eat them every day.

**THE SEVENTH RULE** is to **reduce sugar consumption** and to substitute whole fruit (pineapple, strawberries, etc.) for sugar wherever possible. Sugar or fruit juice causes your body to release too much insulin, which can cause reactive hypoglycemia. This makes you extremely hungry, a condition to avoid when dieting! Also, insulin promotes additional fat storage throughout your body. Use apple butter or apple juice concentrate, but use them in small amounts to avoid reactions.

**THE EIGHTH RULE** would be to **eat frequent meals** or snacks whenever you're hungry - be sure NOT to skip meals. Body fat is burned most efficiently in the presence of carbohydrates and burning the fat properly is comparable to making a fire with the proper wood. Eating meals high in complex carbohydrates regularly also will "spare" body proteins, organs and muscles from being used as fuel. The body prefers to burn glucose from carbohydrates. So don't skip meals, or you will lose body proteins that can be converted to glucose more easily than body fat.

**THE NINTH RULE** is to **exercise** consistently and properly for maximum weight loss. Recent experiments have shown exercises involving the largest muscle groups (legs, hips and back), such as walking, jogging, dancing, using mini-trampolines, stair-steppers, treadmills and exercise bikes, will burn off more fat from the hard-to-lose areas like the stomach, thighs or hips, than will specific exercises like sit-ups and bending motions.

In one important experiment, 13 college men completed 5,004 sit-ups during a 27-day program, averaging about 187 sit-ups daily per person. Each man's fat content was measured both by fat biopsies and water immersion. As we suspected, there was no greater fat loss in the abdominal fat cells than in the fat storage in cells located throughout the body. This means spot reducing (sit-ups or arm exercises) will tone up specific muscles, but will not reduce fat cells in specific areas. So, the best way to burn fat is to do exercises using the largest muscle groups because more total calories will be burned up in a given amount of time.

To burn off the most fat from your stomach, hips or whichever part you're trying to reduce, you should walk, jog, dance, etc. continuously for at least 15 to 60 minutes a day. Although the stomach muscles are too small a group to get maximum fat burning, you should still do toning exercises for all specific muscle groups to keep firm. In addition, it's been found exercising about 30 minutes just before your evening meal will help to reduce your appetite by releasing glycogen (storage glucose). This will help you to burn more fat weight and maintain muscle tone. However, the best time to exercise for most people is in the morning. Studies have shown long term adherence to exercise plan is better for morning exercisers as compared with evening exercisers.

**EXERCISE FOR FITNESS AND FAT LOSS**
**Aerobic** walking with Heavy hands, stair-stepper, jogging, stationary biking for long, slow distances: 15-60 minutes per day, 5-6 days a week. Light weight lifting for muscle toning: 20 minutes, 2 days a week.

**THE TENTH RULE** is to *remain patient.* Don't be discouraged with seemingly slow weight loss. If you had been on a high protein diet, your tissues would have been dehydrated. As you follow **The Healthy Aging Plan,** your muscles will reabsorb vital fluid. Also your body will hold 4 to 10 lb. more bulk food in the intestines. You may believe you're gaining weight during the first month following the program. Actually, you'll be burning fat at the most rapid pace of any program yet developed. Stay on **The Healthy Aging Plan** at least six months and you will appreciate how easily those inches of fat will shrink away, without being hungry. Calorie and portion restricted programs leave you hungry, but on **The Healthy Aging Plan** you can eat tasty, low fat foods whenever you feel slightly empty or hungry. You will always feel good, month after month, which is strong motivation to stay on this plan for life.

Men tend to carry fat weight around the waist area. Women retain fat mostly in the hips, thighs and buttocks. This is a genetic problem that will take about six months to two years to resolve on the best possible program, **The Healthy Aging Plan.** Fat can take months or years to get rid of, which is why you must establish this plan as a way of life. When you lose the fat, by changing your daily eating and exercise habits, you can keep it off for a lifetime. Listen to The Delgado "How to Look and Feel Great" cassette tapes daily for long term motivation, support and instructions. Feeding your mind with positive thoughts will help you to keep on track and achieve your weight loss goal.

**TEN RULES FOR FAT LOSS SUMMARY**
1. Eat more water rich complex carbohydrates.
2. Eat large bowls of soup several times per day.
3. Consume large servings of veggies for lunch, snacks & dinner - salad bar, soups or casseroles.
4. Eat whole fresh fruit (3-8 pieces per day).
5. Reduce fats to less than 22 grams per day.
6. Eat high fiber, low density foods (less grains, more veggies).
7. Reduce sugar (simple carbohydrates).
8. Eat frequent meals whenever you are slightly hungry.
9. Exercise daily (15 to 60 minutes) do aerobics, walk, or jog, etc.
10. Be patient: expect great results in six months to two years.

Follow the ten rules listed above and you will attain your ideal weight. After you've achieved your perfect weight, you may increase your intake of grains, beans, sweet potatoes, breads, uncooked cereals, and reduce the use of vegetables, fruits and wheat bran.

**A Lifetime Diet You can live with**
Why not introduce dieters to **The Healthy Aging Plan** to get the best weight loss, save money, and improve total health? You will be successful in losing weight if you follow **The Healthy Aging Plan,** which encourages you to change your eating habits for a lifetime.

Become knowledgeable and don't be afraid to eat more of the whole natural foods on **The Healthy Aging Plan.** Your friends might lose weight faster initially on their Weight Watcher's or starvation liquid diets, but you will pass them up in a few months and never be fat again, unlike your friends who will always struggle until they also learn **The Healthy Aging Plan.**

You will lose fat weight effectively if you eat less than 20 grams of fat per day and never more than 40 grams. Your total percentage of calories from fat should be under 20%. This is the **Healthy Aging 20-20 rule:** less than 20 grams of fat, under 20% fat to lose fat and keep it off. Your calorie intake will be under 2000, with an average of between 1000 and 1700 calories per day. To keep under 1700 calories per day just be sure to eat generous helpings of soups, fruits, vegetables, potatoes and complex carbohydrates without added fats and sugars. Eat more of the fiber and balanced foods that nature has provided.

Here are the **HEALTHY AGING FOOD GROUPS:**
1. Green vegetables
2. Yellow/orange vegetables
3. Tuber-root vegetables (potatoes, beets, etc.)
4. Citrus and non-citrus fruits
5. Sprouted Grains (two or more types per day)
6. Beans and peas (green, Chinese, split, black-eyed, chick) *or
    B-12 supplements preferably in combination with a B
    complex.
Note: include a weekly serving of sea vegetables (kelp, kombu, wakame, nori) and nuts and seeds for additional trace minerals.

Low fat meats, chicken, fish, turkey, flank steak and nonfat dairy products should only be used as a condiment and never as a main dish (you may choose not to use any meat or dairy product). You should say, "We're having potato pasta casserole," instead of saying, "We're having chicken tonight with a side dish of vegetables."

A 1989 survey by the *California Department of Health* of 1000 consumers discovered that over 25 % of those questioned ate no fruits or vegetables on any given day. Nearly two-thirds of Californians don't eat enough fruits and vegetables. Mass media advertising has led to reliance on fast food burgers, frozen dinners and fatty dairy products. The information in this book will show you how to improve your diet dramatically and gain control over hunger and improper food selections.

# XII

∞

# Exercise for Busy People

---

To have high energy, exercise aerobically for about 30 minutes to an hour every day. You can sustain a pace based on your pulse rate with the formula 20 minus your age x .60 = your target pulse rate to maintain during each session. Also monitor your respiration rate during exercise. You should be able to carry on a conversation during exercise and not get our of breath. If you are out of breath, huffing and puffing then slow down. Your respiration rate is the best way to tell if you are in aerobic exercise.

Some people will do just fine with a brisk walk, slow walk, or jogging. Other exercise we recommend includes a treadmill, stair-master, recline bike, and cross country skiing. Also, weight training at least four times a week for 30 to 45 minutes at high intensity will keep all your muscles fit and in shape. Start with aerobics for 30 minutes and then finish with some weight training.

Busy people may have time for only one session a day. Yet, as we age, muscle tone and strength can be improved if you perform two or three exercise sessions a day. Each exercise session should take less than 30 to 45 minutes. You will be amazed at your rapid progress. Allow for sufficient rest and recovery (about two hours) between exercise sessions. Rest restores enzyme reserves. Excessive exercise without rest may deplete too much of your enzyme stores.

I apply my own principles to my fitness routine by consistently lifting weights at least once or twice a day. I do "fun" aerobics at least four times a week such as dancing, or playing with my children. Aerobics that provides additional benefits such as time with family or social nights out are activities that I look forward to. Because I enjoy the exercise I do, I look forward to doing it on a daily basis. Doing business meetings, family activities, and social events can create challenges. And I am proud to say that even in the busiest of schedules I have been able to continue to improve my fitness level. Age is not something to fear, it is an issue that requires the most advanced program and planning.

Set a goal to exercise twice a day, a minimum of 15 to 30 minutes every morning and again in the evening. If you miss a session, you will at least have gotten in one exercise period a day. Studies show those people who exercise in the morning are more likely to continue exercising one year later, as compared with those who try to exercise in the afternoon or evening.

I always drink two or three glasses of water and I eat a few grapes, an apple, banana or orange just before I start exercising. You must be well hydrated, otherwise you will become fatigued quickly. In addition, I bring water and some fruit with me to the gym during my workout in case I get thirsty. If you drink fluids before, during and after your exercise, you will find your performance and energy improving dramatically.

Do an exercise that is simple and aerobic in nature. It should employ the largest muscle groups of the body (legs or back). You may want to exercise to an aerobic video tape. You can use a mini trampoline, stationary bike, Nordic track, treadmill or stair-stepper. Try out each of these exercises and acquire the necessary equipment to begin your program today.

I have found the **motorized treadmill** to be one of the best overall fat burning and conditioning exercises available. You can purchase a good treadmill with variable speed control for under $500. If your home has adequate space, place the treadmill in front of the television or stereo. If you are overweight, you should exercise at a walking speed of between two and four miles per hour. It is important that you can talk during your exercise without becoming completely out of breath. Slow your pace down until you find the most comfortable rate. It has been shown walking one mile will bum nearly as much fat as running one mile.

The key to optimum conditioning is long, slow distances as opposed to short, intense workouts. Exercising at your "target heart rate" according to so-called fitness guidelines may be causing you to exercise beyond or below your capabilities. Fitness experts may have led you to believe exercise was of no value unless you worked out hard and intense, at a certain target heart rate (220 - age X 65 to 85%). For most people, who are just starting to exercise, a target heart rate of 65-85 % will be too intense, and lead to avoidance of your daily sessions. For long term success, a slower, consistent pace will give you the best results. For example, a target of 50-65% for a 40-year-old would equal 90-117 beats per minute, sustained during exercise. However, if you can carry on a conversation during your exercise, and go a long, slow distance (LSD), then you don't have to monitor your pulse rate.

A **stair-stepper** is another great indoor exercise that is a better conditioner than a **stationary bike** or **mini trampoline**. You will find you can read a book as you step in place on the foot pads. This will help you to lose track of time so that you will exercise for a longer period. However, if you find the stair-stepper too hard and intense, and it leaves you "huffing and puffing", then stay with the more gentle bicycle or trampoline exercise session.

A daily **walking program** of fifteen minutes to one hour a day will bum fat all over your body. If you have a desire to rid yourself of a fat midsection, don't waste time with sit-ups and spot reducing schemes. Lying on a floor and moving your legs is not as effective as moving your whole body upright and supporting your whole weight and walking. Though riding a bike will help those who can't walk, due to knee or ankle problems, it's still not as effective as walking. Here again, don't expect one walk to shed 20 lb. for you. Daily walks, either alone or in addition to other forms of exercise, will have a cumulative effect, and will greatly improve your body's fat-burning capabilities.

**Speed-walking** or race-walking is not only one of the newest ways to get fit, but one of the safest and the best. It trains, shapes and protects the body if you follow two basic rules: 1) Have your lead foot on the ground when your trailing leg pushes off and 2) you must keep your knee straight as your body passes over that leg.  If the knee is kept straight, the pelvis must rotate to the side to allow the moving leg to swing through without throwing the body off balance. This extra rotation helps to strengthen the lower abdominal muscles, the stomach tucked in and the back flat.

These guidelines offer several advantages. Speed-walking has the lowest injury rate of any sport, because the maximum impact per step is about half that of jogging. One foot is always supporting the body and this also makes the walker's stride shorter than a runner's. You also burn more energy to cover the same distance as runner's at the same speed. For example, at 12 minutes per mile, a jogger burns 480 calories per hour and a speedwalker burns 530.

Technique is very important for a good cardiovascular workout, and the better the technique, the faster you'll reshape your body.

1) Start by keeping your back straight and walk tall. This will help you to breathe properly and the high enter of gravity will help give you a full leg extension necessary for a long stride.

2) Point your feet straight and put them at 40 degree angles to the ground. As the edge of your heel hits, tilt your foot to the outside edges of the shoe and lock your ankle. This allows a smooth transition from your heel to your big toe.

3) As you push forward with one leg, push straight back with the other leg until toe-off. As you speed up, try to narrow your stride to get more length and give more stretch to your hips.

4) Concentrate on stretching your hips forward instead of from side to side. Your hips will sway slightly from side to let your trailing leg swing by, but an exaggerated hip wiggle is poor form.

After a few minutes, gradually start to swing your arms. You'll discover you naturally bend your elbows which gives you arms a shorter, faster swinging motion Close your fists loosely and start pumping your arms across your chest. This will free your hips for a longer and faster step.

Start you walking workouts slowly and gradually build up your sessions. Try to do three or four walking workouts, thirty minutes each, every week. Also, experts say walkers should not carry hand weights. They tend to tire the arms quickly and throws you out of synch and disrupt your stride.

You should be able to carry on a conversation without being too short of breath. If speech is difficult and your breathing is labored, you are walking too fast. On the other hand, to get a good aerobic workout, you can't walk too slow. Find a happy medium and this will be the most beneficial.

A consistent program of aerobic exercise also helps to burn fat. When you first begin to workout, your body will burn glucose as its' source of energy. However, over time your body learns to burn fat more efficiently.

Another key to success is to choose a time to walk that is most convenient, so you will be more inclined to follow through. For some people, it is before breakfast, for others it may in the evening after work. Whichever you choose, it is important to pick a time so you will stick with the program.

If it is warm out, take extra precautions to avoid dehydration by drinking water before you begin. Don't use thermal wear, such as pads, etc., because you do risk dehydration with these items. You are not letting your body cool naturally and this can be dangerous.

This aerobic exercise has a purpose to energize your body. If you exercise once in the morning and again in the evening, you will burn fat from your bloodstream. This keeps the blood clearer of triglycerides and helps maintain better circulation. Of course, your diet is very important! You must follow a low fat diet if you expect to be successful. Aerobics also help to build your lung capacity.

Speed-walking is better than long distance, hard jogging. A hard, intense, fast workout is very draining to your body and to the immune system. Your body needs time to recover and intense workouts can hamper your recovery time. Most people end up running too hard, too fast, too long. You can have fun with this type of aerobic workout and still get in good condition.

## AEROBICS
Walk on the treadmill for fifteen minutes to thirty minutes, at three to four and one half miles per hour. This is great for building up the calves. Treadmill work is the ultimate cardiovascular enhancer. Walking one hour after your workout helps with recovery by removing waste from the muscles, while oxygenating the muscles and bloodstream. **Walking also reduces bodyfat more efficiently than other forms of exercises.**

Try stepping on a stair-stepper for fifteen to twenty minutes. The stairs-tepper is great for building up the hips and thighs, and it will build a better cardiovascular base for future workouts. There is now a **portable stair-stepper** that you can take with you in your car, on a vacation, or to the office.

If the work you do during the day requires you to sit for long hours, than doing an upright exercise is going to build-up muscles you don't normally use while sitting. However, if your work requires you to stand for long hours, then it would be better to do exercises like peddling on the **Reclining Bike**, or the regular upright bike. This will allow you to be "off your feet" and it will give your standing muscles a break, while you still get a good cardiovascular effect.

Exercise will strengthen your muscles so that your body will burn fat more efficiently. Mitochondria, the power house of the cells, will increase in number, which will improve your body's ability to bum fat. People who are overweight bum fat less efficiently. By following **The Healthy Aging Plan** of daily exercise and frequent low fat meals, the process of fat-burning can be accomplished easily.

Daily aerobic exercise will help your body's fat cells to release more fat into the bloodstream sooner to be burned by your muscles. This will allow your body to bum more storage fat during and after exercise, instead of burning mostly glucose. Fit people who exercise daily become "fat burners." Unfit people, who are unaccustomed to daily exercise start out burning mainly glucose and not much fat. Your body has two fuel tanks to choose from, one filled with glucose and one filled with fat (unlike your car that has only one fuel tank of gas.) Eventually, after several months of rhythmic, distance exercise your body will select fat as its preferred fuel. This happens because glucose and storage glycogen is used up so quickly that your body will conserve glucose and become conditioned to bum fat. If you follow our low fat diet, there will be almost no fat in your bloodstream, so your body will focus on burning released storage fat from your fat cells as you exercise.

## MUSCLE POWER

In this books, I have described in great detail a plan for nutrition and good health. Here, in this section, "Muscle Power", I will give you the latest information on how to build an outstanding physique, without drugs, in a minimum amount of time.

I've been reading "Muscle & Fitness" magazines, Sports and Fitness research, and medical journals for over twenty-five years! In 1962 I began my first muscle building program inspired by my father, who gave me my first set of "iron" weights (which I still own to this day). By 1966, I began following the careers of Arnold Swartzeneggeer, and Franco Columbo. In 1973 I began "high intensity" training described by Mike Mentzer, Casey Viator, and Arthur Jones (the developer of Nautilus). In 1992 I started experimenting with the Bulgarian method of training.

All the training concepts differed. Each program contradicted the others. Some argued that fast repetitions were best, others said super-slow repetitions worked better. Some said, use "negative" eccentric contractions, others said no, use "positive" concentric contractions. Some said train frequent long hours, others said train short, brief intense periods of time, etc. Who was right?

Arthur Jones did an experiment with identical twins and he had one do negative reps (letting the weight down, lengthening the muscle fibers) and the other do only positive reps (lifting the weight up, shortening the muscle fibers). The negative reps built the most strength and size, according to my training partner, Brian Sutton. Add brief intense sessions, done more frequent, to give additional benefit.

I had studied muscle structure, human anatomy and physiology at Physical Therapy school in the Masters program at USC. I learned about nutrition and medical research at the Pritikin Longevity Center, under my mentor, Nathan Pritikin from 1979 to 1981. It was Nathan Pritikin who taught me to question all so called "truths," and to look for the "real truth."

University courses always seem behind the times. To this day, I continually review medical journals and study with the "top people" in their respective fields, looking for better ways to build the mind, body, and spirit. To build my spirit and mind I have turned to the teachings of Tony Robbins, Zig Ziglar, Wayne Dyer, Brian Tracy, and, The Bible.

I knew that almost all the world's top athletes and bodybuilders were using dangerous anabolic growth drugs to build-up their physiques. I personally refused to take "steroids", or anything artificial or drug related. So I have continually looked for safe, effective, natural ways to build strength and vitality.

In 1979 the Bulgarians started a revolution in muscle building. Later, they took the leading role in the weight lifting events in the Olympics. They beat the Russians, the Cubans, and the Americans. No one knew their training secrets, until very recently.

The Bulgarians workout more often in a day, than some athletes workout in a week. They are able to workout three to seven times a day, because each session is shorter (less than forty-four minutes each workout). Also, each workout is intense, using heavy weights with progressive increases.

The more frequent, **brief, intense workouts,** you do in a **day,** the more your muscles will adapt to the continual irritation and stimulation, to build bigger, and stronger muscles.

The success of an athlete in this type of intense, frequent, training routine will depend on his or her adaptive energies. Recovery after workouts to build muscle is dependent on adaptive energies.

You can increase the intensity and productivity of your workouts by focusing your mind on powerful thoughts. Visualize a powerful image such as a volcano exploding, or a rocket ship taking off as you press the weight. See yourself projecting this flow of energy past the end of your arms beyond the bar.

Initially, you might feel tired and weak, from exercising more often. However, be encouraged because you will continue to progress with each workout. Your body will adapt to higher levels of training, heavier weights, and more frequent workouts, as each day of training is completed.

Now you may ask, how can you shape your body to fit your desired outcome? The fact is that THE ENERGY SYSTEM you use most often DETERMINES your BODYSHAPE. If you use the Lactic Acid energy system, you will have larger, fuller muscles like a bodybuilder. If you use the ATP-PC energy system, you will have a thick, dense power-lifter look. If you use the Aerobic energy system, you will look slender, like a distance runner with a lower body fat level.

Your genetic makeup or individual potential to build muscle is in large part determined by your parents or grandparents. For example, you may have noticed the calve muscles, biceps, or forearms of a father and his son are almost identical in shape and size. However, you can reach your full genetic potential by the type of training you do daily.

Your body will adapt faster and increase in strength, if you train first with the idea to build more muscular size. As your muscles get bigger, your potential to build more strength will become greater.

**Aerobic exercise as compared to Anaerobic exercise**
You probably have heard of "aerobic exercises" (long, slow, distances) and "anaerobic exercises" (short, fast, movements).

The anaerobic exercises can be done without oxygen. Running sprints and weight lifting are examples of exercises that employee anaerobic metabolism.

Our bodies can use two different types of anaerobic energy systems. One is the lactic acid, and the other is the ATP-PC. The lactic acid energy system is employed when you are doing an exercise that burns up glucose so rapidly that an oxygen debt develops. This will leave a byproduct of lactic acid to be used for energy as needed.

In the past, we thought of lactic acid as just a waste product that we had to try to clear from our systems, as soon as possible. However, we now know that in trained athletes, lactic acid can be used as a very efficient and powerful fuel.

When your goal is to gain muscular weight, you should keep your training focused on using the lactic acid energy system. Growth hormones are produced and released into the bloodstream during lactic acid energy system training.

1) The lactic acid energy system is employed if your lifting weights that are between 65% and 90% of your maximum lift for the particular exercise you are doing. For example, if you could normally lift 200 pounds in the bench press for one repetition, than you would use between 130 and 180 pounds during a set of five to fifteen repetitions. The rest between sets should

stay between 30 seconds for smaller muscles like the biceps, and up to three minutes for larger muscles of the legs or back. **Shorter rests of less than three minutes between sets, will allow you to perform more sets for each body part per session. Doing high volume training where you perform the maximum number of sets (15 to 18) in 30 to 40 minutes will add the most size. Just allow enough rest to perform the next set with maximum effort. This type of training will release the maximum amount of growth hormones.**

This release of growth hormones occurs within fifteen minutes after a workout. If you workout in this manner at least one to three times a day you will produce more growth hormones and make rapid progress. This will make your body build bigger muscles. This is the type of training used by successful bodybuilders. If you do this type of training you will have larger, fuller muscles and look more like a bodybuilder.

You still should do some training using the Adenosine Triphosphate (ATP) and Creatine Phosphate (PC) energy system.

**2)** Your body uses this ATP-PC energy system to build strength with short, intense bursts of maximal lifts. You would use a weight that would be between 90 and 100% of maximum during a set of between one and three repetitions. In the example above of the bench press, you would lift between 180 and 200 pounds for one to three repetitions, if 200 pounds was the maximum you could lift for one lift.

Also, you would rest longer periods between sets, at least three minutes to five minutes or more between sets. This will allow for full recovery of the muscles to perform another maximal lift and total replacement of glucose in the muscles being worked. This type of training is used by power lifters, Olympic lifters, and wrestlers. If you primarily do this type of training you will have thick, dense, strong muscles.

When you want to reduce body fat, and condition the cardiovascular system, you will need to do additional aerobic exercises.

**3)** The aerobic energy system of the body is used when you go for long, slow distance walks or jogs. It should take between twenty minutes to an hour to cover two to five miles. You should be able to carry on a conversation during the exercise without being too out of breath. This is the training system used primarily by marathon runners. If this is the only type of training you do, long, slow distances, then you will look like a marathon runner.

Remember, you can have the best of all worlds and develop the look and training effect you want. Now you have it, you can build up muscular size, strength, and aerobic fitness, by using these different training concepts. However, now we need to go into more details to insure your success.

To achieve maximal muscular growth, you must train, train, train! The more you train the more you build muscle. Eating more protein will not force muscular growth. Good nutrition centered on complex carbohydrates will allow for quicker recovery after the workouts. Complex carbohydrate foods like sprouted bread, brown rice, and yams provide high quality energy and protein to spare body proteins and allow for the maximum anabolic growth of muscles and the least amount of catabolism (breakdown of muscular tissue).

*The New England Journal of Medicine, Oct. 5, 1989* showed that frequent snacks eaten every hour (17 meals in a day!) as compared to the same foods and calories eaten only three times in a day dramatically reduced the urine output of cortisol by nearly 20%.

This last point of a reduction in cortisol output is of great significance to bodybuilders and athletes. You see, cortisol is the most potent catabolic agent. Cortisol is a substance that rapidly breaks down muscle tissue and reduces muscular size and strength. The cortisol substance is naturally released into the bloodstream and circulates in the bloodstream after weight training. This means that eating frequent meals, especially meals high in complex carbohydrates, can have a dramatic anti-catabolic effect.

Normally, bodybuilders rely on steroids to clear cortisol from the circulation. But, the moment the athlete stops using steroids, there will be a rapid build-up of cortisol that can continue to breakdown the muscles for over a six-month period. This is one reason their muscular size shrinks back down so quickly after stopping steroid abuse. This recent discovery, that eating more frequent meals can reduce the catabolic effect, could be one way to reduce the dependency on steroids. Steroids also have an anabolic effect (building-up muscle), but only if intense weight training is done to stimulate muscular growth. This same anabolic effect (muscle build-up) will occur from weight training by itself. Certainly not as dramatic as with steroid use, however, muscle building can be more permanent and long lasting, without dangerous side effects. So the **key** to more muscular growth is to consume frequent meals high in carbohydrates and to train at least 5 times a week, heavy and intense.

The feeling you should have from training is a constant dull ache in the muscles. You will find that a continual feeling of muscle soreness, and muscle fatigue will lead to the maximum in muscular growth and strength. According to the Bulgarians, if you feel strong and powerful for more than three days, you are probably not providing sufficient irritation and stimulation to the muscles to promote growth!

As you workout more often, one or two times a day with more intensity, you will notice at times you feel weaker. This temporary weakness is a good sign, because as you persist with frequent daily workouts you will soon be making great gains. As you continue, stay encouraged and confident even though you may experience temporary dips in strength, and size, because after about the fourth or fifth week of this type of training and feeling you will rebound and skyrocket in size and strength.

Don't get discouraged. If you listen to your body, you will be convinced to take a day off and rest. Don't stop. Don't skip a workout just because you don't feel strong. Be your own coach. A coach would push you even when you want to give-up. You always can squeeze out just a little bit more, even after you thought you gave 100% effort. Follow the plan I'm about to lay out for you and you will see fantastic improvements.

At this point you need to ask yourself an important question. Is your current exercise program consistent with the outcome you want? Realistically, if you're a professional or Olympic athlete then going through the "pain and the discomfort" of heavy weight training will help to achieve your goal. To an athlete, it is worth the sacrifice to delay gratification, be disciplined, work hard, and put up with some discomfort, because their very livelihood is dependent on it. As an athlete, you must be willing to pay the price, and you need to know what it will take to develop the ultimate in power, strength, and fitness.

However, to the housewife who wants to have a more shapely, attractive body, look better, have more energy, and feel strong, she can accomplish these goals quickly and efficiently with less effort than that of an athlete. You will need to modify and apply this information to fit your needs. The extent to which you apply these principals, will give you the results you want.

Two important things I learned from Arnold Swartzeneggeer and Mike Mentzer was to train hard and to focus on the task at hand. I also learned how important it is to rest just before important events.

There are three important levels of recovery our bodies go thorough during exercise programs: acute, intermediate, and long-term recovery. Acute recovery that takes only about two to **five minutes**, and it occurs between sets of weight lifting as your heart rate slows back down, and your muscles restore ATP and remove waste products.

The second level of recovery is called intermediate recovery. It takes one to two hours for the body to restore blood glucose and hormone levels back to normal after a workout.

Long term recovery can take seven days or more, and this is measured by your total body energy, strength levels, and how you "feel."

Arnold would diet and workout hard all year, and then he would stop weight training just days before a bodybuilding contest. This would give his muscles a chance to grow to their peak of development. The rest would allow him to regain his strength, and feel powerful before he stepped up on stage to flex his muscles and to perform.

Now let's go back to more of these new weight training and exercise principals. By applying these concepts, you to can experience a powerful feeling and gain muscular development like you never have before.

## NEW TRAINING PRINCIPLES
The speed that you do the set is of major importance. Each repetition should be done as with force and controlled while you move the weight. Lift the weight fast, without swinging the weight. Try to prevent momentum from taking over. The faster you lift the weight the greater the intensity, and stimulating irritation to the muscles. Start the set with strict form, performing

the lift as fast as possible. When you find the weight moving slower, as you progress into the set, loosen up your form so that you can continue to move the weight as fast as possible. As you find a break in the smooth rhythmic pace of the lift, pause a moment, take a deep breath and then work hard to complete the last two or three repetitions.

Choose a weight that you can barely lift for the number of repetitions called for. If you're supposed to do between five and fifteen repetitions and the particular set your doing calls for 10 reps, then the eleventh rep could not be done if it were attempted. We will outline later how many reps you are to do with each new week of workouts. For now, just remember, begin each set with a weight that you can do with strict form, fast. When the repetitions become impossible to do, "loosen-up" your form to continue the set to completion. Loosen-up your form refers to allowing a slight bounce off the top of the thighs (if you were doing curls) and a slight backward lean as the weight is coming up. This allows you to continue to finish the set.

If a training partner were present, they could assist you with the weight slightly, as the set gets harder to lift. This technique is called a "forced rep."

The set is completed when no further repetitions can be done in reasonable form. This is known as "relative maximum voluntary muscular contraction." Every set must be done to this point, just before momentary muscular failure, to achieve maximum muscular growth. It's psychologically important to make each rep. Experienced lifters can feel this point just before failure, without continuing to actual failure. This is the stage during the set when your form is beginning to loosen and the pace of the movement is getting slower.

There are ways to extend the set using six different methods that will increase the intensity of your workouts. These methods should only be used in some sets, and in some of your workouts. If used every time, and every set, it can cause you to experience problems of over-training and burnout. This could deplete your adaptive energies, and slow your total progress.

1. **Descending sets** or pyramiding - As you reach momentary exhaustion in a set, quickly, without rest, select a lighter weight and do a few more reps. Or select a heavier weight midway through your set, and finish with fewer reps, but with a heavier weight.

2. **Partial Reps** - Finish your set with several partial reps with the same weight. Do this at the point where you can no longer complete a full movement with the weight, however, you still can do shorter peak contraction sets, as with curls.

3. **Negative Reps** - At the completion of the set, do "eccentric movements" as you let the weight down, you are always stronger, and can do a few more reps. You need a training partner for this one, or a free hand for dumbbell curls to help the weight up to let the weight back down. Hydraulic weights, where you control the weight, or nautilus foot pedals work in a similar fashion, to allow you to lift the weight up easier, and leave a heavier amount of weight to fight on the downward descent. Your muscles are stronger on the downward descent in letting a weight down "eccentric" (when the muscle fibers lengthen) as opposed to lifting the weight up "concentric" contractions (when the muscle fibers shorten).

4. **Giant set** - As you complete a set, you are to begin immediately performing another exercise that works the same muscle. For example, you might start with a set of curls, and then do pulldowns with no rest between sets. The curls pre-exhaust the biceps, and the pulldowns still work the biceps, and with the aid of the lats (back muscle), you can work the biceps past exhaustion. Giant sets will increase the intensity or stimulation being focused on the biceps in this case. This will induce more growth and strength to develop in the biceps.

5. **Forced Reps** - Were described above - your partner gives you just enough help to complete the last few reps.

6. **Cheating Reps** - also described above, where you "loosen up" your form, then can cheat two or three more reps out of the set.

NOTE - Supersets are not as effective and not to be used. This is where you train a different body part with no rest between sets, i.e., bench press with stomach crunches. This may give you a "pump", however you're only opening up blood vessels to more blood, but you're not allowing for enough rest between sets, and you're not working the individual muscles hard enough.

"Free weights" are best to use during compound movements involving several muscle groups like those in the back, or legs.

The "machine weights" are best for isolation single muscle (biceps, triceps etc.) exercises. Ideally, 70% of your training should be with "Free Weights."

The Bulgarians made an amazing discovery regarding the ideal length of time to train for each session. Blood samples taken during workouts showed that we should train between 35 and 44.5 minutes to maintain the highest natural testosterone levels. If you train past 45 minutes, your testosterone levels can drop over 80%. This means that though your desire and motivation to train past 45 minutes is still driving you, your natural anabolic hormone level is very low. Therefore, your ability to recover and build up muscle is always best if you train less than 44 minutes per session!

This shorter training session, also allows you to keep higher glucose levels for ATP production and storage, for your next high energy workout. And you will find that you can keep your mental focus higher, so that you can look forward to your next short workout.

Atrophy of muscle begins within 72 hours of the last workout. Therefore, each muscle part must be trained at least every three days (72 hours). The Bulgarians found that we can train the same muscle group again within 45 minutes after the last session. This proves that recovery following workouts occurs much faster than we previously thought. This allows you the opportunity to train each body part more frequently without the risk of over-training. Once you realize this, you can train more often each day, and accelerate your rate of muscular growth. Ideally, train each muscle group at least three times a week.

The Bulgarians lacked fear of over-training. They discovered the body's true capabilities. The two most effective things you can do to increase your muscular size and strength is to train each body part more frequently and to reduce the time of each training session.

The Bulgarians start their athletes out at 11 and 12 years of age training three to four times each day. As their physical ability progresses, they begin to train four to seven times a day. These are short, intense workout sessions, done several times a day.

Now I know what your thinking. Are you nuts, I don't have time to train three to seven times a day!! But, you know what? The moment you realize this new potential, you will stop limiting yourself. It's just like running the four minute mile. Once Roger Banister broke the record, though everyone thought it was humanly impossible to run that fast, hundreds of other runners broke the record as well. It was a mental barrier, not a physiological human potential barrier.

This motivated me to set up my weight room at my office at work. I also dusted off my weights at home. I began going to the gym more often. After only 21 days I began noticing improvements where I couldn't improve before. I broke through plateau's and I began to stretch myself mentally and physically. It's been fun and I look forward to my training sessions. Some days I work two training sessions into my day. Some days, I play basketball with my son Jason. Other days, I only get in a walking session. Yet it still is working for me, and by striving to workout every day, I average about four to five sessions a week.

## FINAL SUMMARY TIPS TO BUILD MUSCLE:

* Workout at least **once a day**. On weekends or during the week, if time permits workout **two times a day**. Working out **two times a day will give you your most rapid gains in muscularity and in strength**.
* **Rest** at least **one** to **two hour** between workouts.
* Workouts should last only **thirty-five** to **forty-four minutes** to maintain high testosterone levels. Remember, if you workout with weights past forty-four minutes your testosterone levels will drop rapidly).
* The number of repetitions, number of sets, rest between sets, and type of exercises should vary.
* You should workout in cycles of three weeks, and then change your routine.
* Divide the bodyparts to be trained per day into the different muscle groups.
   Start out your program by working out about once or twice a day. It is best to build a base with only one or two sessions per day for about eighteen weeks to get you into condition for later workouts of four or five times a week..

## ADVANCED TRAINING PROGRAM
   You can use the following training routine that I have developed and found to be effective. Each session is divided into what I call a "blast". Exercises

179

are divided into "push" sessions and "pull" sessions.

Start with "blast number one" - **pushing exercises**, working on the shoulders, chest, triceps and thighs. An entire blast session can be done in 25 to 45 minutes. Take a set of dumbbells with a weight that allows you to do 3 sets of **shoulder flys**:

Arms extended, bend forward at the waist and do two sets lifting the weights out to your side, like you are flying. Next, do two sets of shoulder fly's while standing straight. Complete the last set by holding the dumbbells straight in front of your and lifting them up and down your full range of motion.

You will complete your shoulder work with two sets of military press divided behind the neck and two sets in front of your neck. As you lift the barbell straight over head, you are working your shoulders, trapezius and triceps. However, because you worked shoulder fly's first, the military press will stimulate the deltoid (shoulder muscles) and work them harder than the other muscle groups. An effective technique to build the deltoids even more is to first do a set of shoulder fly's followed quickly by a set of military press.

**Chest** is the next pushing exercise to perform. You should isolate the pectoralis major and minor chest muscles by first doing five sets of butterfly's at different angles. Lie on an incline bench, flat bench and declined bench. Hold the dumbbells out at your sides and bring the weight together in an arch and back down. Chest work continues with 1 to 3 sets of bench press. The bench press uses multiple muscle groups (chest, shoulders, triceps). This allows deeper penetration to muscle fibers that take more intense work before they will begin working. During my chest workout, I will sometimes "pre-exhaust" the chest muscle fibers with a set of butterfly's, followed immediately (no rest period) by a set of bench press. This will cause all the muscle fibers of the chest to work at full capacity. This creates maximum stimulation of deep muscle fibers not normally worked.

**Triceps** (back of your arms) can be exercised with cable extensions, body dips and tight grip bench press.

**Thighs** can be exercised with leg extensions, followed by leg presses and squats.

"Blast number two" uses **pulling exercises** (back, biceps, hamstrings, calves, abdominal.) Your **back** can be worked best by doing Nautilus pullovers and cable rows. I have a cable belt that straps around the middle of my arms. This removes the action of the biceps and allows more direct work on the back muscles. I like to work the back with at least three different exercises (pullovers, rows and pulldowns). Do 3 sets each for a total of 9 sets. I do pull-ups and pull-downs (LAT machine with cables) last. This naturally leads into biceps work. The pull-down automatically works the latisimus dorsi, as well as the biceps.

The **biceps** can now be worked with heavy curls, preacher curls on the Scott bench, followed by single arm Nautilus curls. When you do single arm curls (with Nautilus or a dumbbell), you can weight up slightly as the set progresses.

**Hamstrings** (back of the legs) can be worked with a Flexion machine with three to five sets. **Calves** will gain from calf raises and walking or running.

**Abdominal** and stomach muscles are small. They can be effectively worked with 2 sets of 12 repetitions divided between knee-bent quarter sit-ups, crunches and leg lifts.

"Blast number three" can include **leg** adduction (leg pull together), abduction (legs push apart), hip flexion (Nautilus machine works hips and gluteus maximus effectively), and the Stair-stepper machine (leaning back works the hips and buttock muscles.) Finish with full leg driving squats. Cool down with a walking aerobic session.

You can "blast" three times a weed and work the full body, virtually every muscle, in one week. Each blast should be short - 25 to 45 minutes, with at least one day rest between each blast. Blast in sequential order: number one, two, three and start your next session with number one again on the same day or on another day. Don't worry if you miss a session or two. You will make excellent progress if you workout three to four times a week. However, if you only workout three a week, you can still prevent muscular atrophy and loss of muscular tone. If you just want to stay in shape, then do blast one, two and three once a week (M, W, F) with daily aerobics done thirty to one hour a day.

As you workout from month to month, you should vary the number of sets, repetitions, types of exercise and combinations of exercises done during a blast session. This will help you to avoid sticking points and boredom. Muscles need constant stimulation. If your goal is to gain muscular weight, you must workout heavy, fast and frequently (at least three times a day.)

After you have completed the last routine of training, you can repeat the cycle from the very beginning. Ideally, you should change your type of workout every three weeks. The number of times you train per day is up to you. Your schedule, your goals, and your progress will help you to establish the proper routine. Keep a prospective on fitting your exercise into your daily schedule. Maintain a balance, and enjoy your exercise as part of your life. The quality of your life will be enhanced immeasurably, as you age gracefully with strength and vitality.

The above is just an example of training routines you can do. Maybe some weeks you'll have more time and you can train two or three times in a day. But, try to train at least once a day. Remember, if you miss a few days of training, your still ahead of the game. Because training four times a week, will still bring you progress, and keep you in shape. Muscles start to atrophy in 72 hours (three days)! So, if you try to train only four days a week and you miss a few workouts, you will need to get back into a consistent routine.

Sometimes you may decide to miss days of exercise because your body became stressed from "over-training." Signs of over-training include an elevation of your pulse of 8 to 10 beats per minute above your normal morning resting pulse. Also, an elevation of your systolic* blood pressure (the higher number -120* over 80) of 10 mm Hg or more over your normal level. Other signs of over-training can include loss of appetite, loss of interest in training, inability to relax, depression, or swelling of lymph nodes in the neck, groin, or armpits.

If signs of over-training should develop, just switch to a simple walking program for a week or two, and you will recover quickly.

The key is to expand your mind, and train as often as possible, within the limits of your genetic capabilities. Now make room in your schedule to exercise and get started today. You can do it. So get started and just do it!

# XIII

∞

# How to Look Great by Shrinking Your Fat Cells and Increase Your Energy

---

**The Healthy Aging Diet and Exercise Plan** is designed so that anyone can stay on it for a lifetime. Women can develop and maintain that new attractive figure, a leaner body with a firm abdomen, curvaceous hips and a radiant face with the cheeks of a model. Men will have a muscular, firm, better-proportioned appearance. You will get compliments from men and women who remember your past struggles with starvation and food restriction diets. Failure, pain, hunger and weakness can all be turned into success, pain free satisfaction and energy on **The Healthy Aging Plan.**

Women need fat, but in the right places - distributed evenly over the body for a smooth, soft look. For example, a 130 lb., 5'4" ideally proportioned woman, participating in daily exercise classes and capable of running a 26-mile marathon may have 15% body fat. Therefore, 15 to 20% body fat would be a lean, athletic, well-shaped woman. The breakdown of fat distribution may be as follows: 2 - 4 lb. for breasts, 4 lb. of fat in the intestinal area, 4 - 5 lb. under the skin and 5 lb. of fat on the back of each thigh. There is also a need in both men and women for about 15 - 30 lb. of essential body fat in the organs and for insulation.

Men look their best when the body fat level is between 5-17%. In 1978 when I was overweight, Dr. Bob Girandola of U.S.C. measured my body fat. He used the water immersion method and my body fat level measured over 25%. He told me I was classified as obese! However, after less than 5 months on my low fat, high carbohydrate diet, with exercise, my weight had reduced from over 200 lb. to 159 lb. Dr. Girandola repeated the test on body fat 4 months after the first test and was amazed that I had reduced to under 9%.

Selecting the right foods for your caloric needs is an effective way to reduce body fat and look years younger. Excess fat leaves a puffy, grotesque look (fatty stomach, hips and face) that makes people look years older.

One study has shown that when subjects were given extra fat added to a low calorie diet, 33% of the fat went right to the fat storage cells. It was discovered by using radioactive tracers placed on the fat in the diet that the fat was stored instead of being used for fuel. The body is not capable of burning more than a certain amount of fat from the diet. The excess will simply be absorbed and stored by the billions of fat cells of the body. Fat storage cells (adipose tissue) act like billions of small sponges. Excess fat from your diet is absorbed by these fat cells daily, even if you are consuming fewer calories.

Your body receives most of its needed fuel for energy (over 80%) from carbohydrates that break down into glucose. Fat is a secondary fuel that can only be used at a constant slow rate. If you remove carbohydrates from a low calorie diet, your body will continue to burn the same constant rate of fat; however, the rest of your caloric needs will come from glucose stored in your liver and muscles. This stored glucose amounts to less than 12 hours of fuel. After 12 hours of avoiding carbohydrate foods, your entire body storage of glucose will be depleted. When this happens, your body then will quickly begin breaking down your muscle proteins into glucose for fuel, instead of burning more fat. This is why the best diet for you should be very low in fat and high in complex carbohydrates, not just low in calories. Your body can only release more fat from the cells than it stores if there is less fat in your diet and more complex carbohydrates.

Fat provides 9 calories per gram, whereas carbohydrate and protein have only 4 calories per gram. This means fat is twice as fattening as any other nutrient.

We all have different capacities to retain or lose fat. Every day that you eat low fat foods and exercise fifteen to sixty minutes, you will be establishing a pattern of success. Month after month you will see your results improving as your fat cells shrink. The actual number of fat cells we have is influenced by three critical periods of time during our lives.

The first comes before birth, during the last three months of pregnancy. If your mother was led to believe good nutrition meant eating more eggs, cheese, milk, butter and meat, then the excessive amount of fat and calories would have stimulated an increase in the number of fat cells in the fetus. If your mother had followed a Healthy Aging type of nutritional plan with whole grain rice, bread, pastas, beans, peas, fruits and vegetables without added fat, you may have developed fewer fat cells.

The next critical period of fat cell development occurs during the first year of life. If your mother gave you high fat (bottle) formulas and introduced fat and sugar-laden foods, then the fat cells would have increased beyond the expected number. Fat cells could double or triple during the first year after birth. However, if you were breast fed, then your body would have produced fewer fat cells.

In the final, critical period, which is during childhood and youth, the fat cells grow both in size and number. Another significant increase because of hormonal changes (puberty for teenage girls) and a fatty diet follow this.

However, if you did develop a large number of fat cells, for any of the above reasons, there is no need to be discouraged. **The Healthy Aging Plan** will slim down the size of your fat cells.

It may take several months or even a full year or two to get to your goal of ideal body weight. However, if you consider that this plan will enable you to achieve a fat free body permanently, it's worth the wait, isn't it?

**Supplements to aid in Fat burning:** Black Walnut, Lecithin, Chitosan, erythorbic acid, citric acid, cruciferous concentrate, Gymena slyvestre, Chromium, Bayberry bark, catnip, chickweed, fenugreek, gentian, golden seal, myrrh, bule vervain, comfrey, prickly ash, St. John Wort, yellow dock, cyani, evening primrose, mandrake, pumpkin seed, wormwood, cloves, sage, garlic, tansy leaves, diatomaceous earth and chlorophyll.

# How To Increase Your Energy

One of the key reasons people participate in **The Healthy Aging Plan** is to increase their energy levels. The complex carbohydrates are your best source of energy. Fat provides you with less quality energy. Protein would be the least acceptable energy source and cause the most fatigue. To have more energy, therefore, eat at least ten servings of vegetables, fruit, and potatoes a day. Use only whole sprouted grains high in complex carbohydrates and take quality supplements.

   Plan ahead, carry food with you in a sack lunch, ice chest or a Cool Tote as I carry with me. This will maintain even glucose levels, giving you a high energy level. The moment you begin to feel weak, an empty stomach or hungry, go ahead and eat lightly. Frequent small meals of complex carbohydrates will be digested into glucose at a slow, consistent rate. Big, heavy meals tend to lead to a build-up of fat in the blood known as triglycerides.

**Triglycerides** are the way fats are carried in the blood and are stored in your fat cells. Pinch the fat on your body and you are pinching triglycerides. To experience high energy, you must maintain low fat levels in your blood. Strive to keep your triglycerides levels under 100 mg and total lipids ideally under 500 at all time during the day, especially after eating.

   Fasting for blood tests have misled people and physicians into ignoring poor dietary habits. By eating frequent, small meals that are low in fat, you can maintain low fat levels in your blood all day and night. This will allow for excellent circulation. The red blood cells will flow freely to carry the maximum amount of oxygen to your brain and all the cells of your body. One fatty meal can cause the blood to become sticky, resulting in clumping of the red blood cells for over 9 hours. If less oxygen reaches the brain, you will become sleepy and tired. This is probably why so many people drink coffee (caffeine is a drug stimulant) to try to stay awake and alert. However, by maintaining low fat triglycerides and total lipids you will experience an incredible increase in energy as more oxygen reaches your brain.

The following steps are necessary to reduce fat in your blood:

**1.** Avoid all oils: polyunsaturated like corn oil, safflower oil, etc., monounsaturated like canola oil, olive oil, etc., and saturated fats found in butter, cheese, red meat, etc.

**2.** Avoid excessive use of sugar, alcohol, fruit juice or dried fruit. Sugars convert into fats if used beyond your caloric needs. Sugars are devoid of fiber so they rush into your bloodstream too quickly and turn into fats.

**3.** Maintain your ideal weight - obesity can cause high fat levels in the blood. In order to have more energy, you must achieve your ideal body weight. If you are currently overweight, choosing all the recommended foods and exercising daily, you may not begin to experience high energy levels until you reach your ideal body weight. If you are carrying 10 to 40 extra pounds on your body and that extra weight is in the form of fat that can enter your bloodstream at any time and slow you down, just as if you had eaten fat. You can reach your ideal body weight by following the recommendations we offer in this book.

**4.** Exercise daily to maintain good circulation and low fat levels. Daily exercise will begin to fire up your system to give you more energy. If you do the minimum of 15 minutes a day that is fine. But why not plan to do 15 minutes in the morning and 15 minutes more at night? By exercising in the morning, you will burn fats that have accumulated during the night while you were sleeping and inactive. Since your triglycerides will be lower, you will have more energy throughout the day. Then at the end of the day, when there is a tendency to have a slight elevation of triglycerides, exercising again for 15 minutes will reduce the fatty levels in your bloodstream. If you want to maintain high energy levels all day long, avoid excessive or intensive exercise. Long, slow distance exercises (walking, swimming, light weights) are better than fast, overly demanding runs and heavy weight training sessions. If you are an athlete or you are accustomed to intense workouts, anticipate a need for several additional hours of sleep to allow your body to recover each day. Training to the point of muscular failure on every exercise is terribly taxing to your energy levels. Start your exercise plan slow. Be consistent and you will look forward to each day with excitement and vigor. If you find yourself avoiding exercise sessions, you probably have been training too hard.

**5.** Reduce stress by focusing on the good things in people and in life. If adrenaline builds up, it can increase blood fats for several hours.

Have your triglycerides, cholesterol and total lipids checked every three weeks until you can maintain ideal levels on a regular basis. After consecutive low readings, you can check your levels every three months to be sure you're still on the right track.

Make sure you get enough sleep each night. Most of our participant's notice they require much less sleep as they eat more raw vegetables, sprouts, fruit, less fat and exercise. You should feel rested and good in the morning without needing coffee, tea or cokes all day. A thirty-minute nap during the day may be beneficial for people who work long hours (12 to 16 hours a day.)

Your physiology, posture, stance and walk are also important to feel energetic. If you slump and slouch you will feel tired. Try sitting up straight and erect and you will notice an immediate improvement. Tony Robbins taught me the importance of frequent aerobic exercise that causes deep breathing, deep breathing sessions, massage and "peak state" sessions to maintain high energy.

Some people suffer from "chronic fatigue syndrome", which can be caused by a number of different conditions. See a doctor to check your thyroid, blood counts, B-12 and iron for anemia, possible viral conditions like Epstein-Barr, mono, etc., allergies and other metabolic diseases like cancer. **The Healthy Aging Plan** can serve as a cornerstone to enhance treatment and in many cases provide full recovery from various energy robbing diseases.

**Supplements that increase energy and endurance:** Alfalfa, Bee Pollen, Cayenne, DHEA, Melatonin, Growth Hormone, Licorice, Siberian Ginseng, Stevia, Suma, Una de Gato, Vitamin B Comples, CoQ10, Garliv, Parsley, Capsicum, Gotu Kola, Missouri snake root, chickweek, guar gum, cascara agrada, red clover, echinacea root, fennel, black walnut, dandelion root and Pyruvate(found in red apples and other foods, however it's better absorbed as a supplement).

# XIV

∞

# Nutrition for Pregnant & Lactating Women, Infants, Children and Teenagers

## PREGNANCY

During pregnancy and while nursing, all the nutritional requirements needed for mother and child are available in the whole, natural foods. The "Healthy Aging Six" food groups provide the best possible sources for energy and nourishment. The six groups are to be eaten in the following order to insure sufficient calories will be consumed:

**1. Sprouted Whole Grains** (a variety of multigrain, and sprouted grains such as spelt, wheat, oats, rice, millet) eaten several times daily.
**2. Beans and Peas**
**3. Tuber Root Vegetables** (Yams, Sweet Potatoes, Potatoes, Beets, Rutabagas).
**4. Citrus, and Non-Citrus Fruits**
**5. Green Vegetables**
**6. Yellow/Orange Vegetables**

**Rice, soy, or almond milk** must be used instead of other **dairy products.**

**Meats, fish, or fowl** should only be used as a **condiment or not eaten at all by using bean and grain substitute meats.**

You also will want to include other vitamin and mineral rich food such as sea vegetables, small amounts of nuts and lots of "sprouted" seeds for additional trace minerals. Be sure to include a daily source of Vitamin B-12, fortified in cereal, or in supplemental form.

The pregnant or lactating woman needs sufficient amounts of these six types of nutrients to nourish her body and her baby:

1. **CARBOHYDRATES -raw food rich in enzymes**
2. **FATS-essential fatty acids from sprouted flaxseed, avocados etc.**
3. **PROTEIN- from sprouted beans, sprouted whole grains**
4. **VITAMINS & MINERALS**
5. **ENZYMES, HERBS**
6. **PURE ORGANIC WATER from FRUITS & VEGETABLES**

**Carbohydrates and fats** provide energy or calories. This "fuel" is necessary for the body to "work" at muscle contraction, nerve impulse conduction, hormone production, wound repair, cell growth, etc. Of course, this is also extremely important in the development of the baby. Grains, potatoes, vegetables, fruits, nuts, seeds and pastas all provide the mother with fuel for energy. On the other hand, animal fats will be stored in the body's fat storage and not burn as efficiently.

**Proteins** are the "building blocks" for muscles, hormones, hair, fingernails, blood, antibodies and of the baby. These individual building blocks are called amino acids and are found in grains, legumes, green vegetables, yams, potatoes, and sprouted seeds. Preeclampsia (high blood pressure and fluid retention) or "toxemia of pregnancy" has been attributed to insufficient protein intake and "empty calorie foods." Therefore, the grains, legumes, etc., all contain high quality protein to fill the body's needs. The "Southern Medical Journal" reported in 1987, a study on 775 pure vegan women (totally meat and dairy free diet) giving birth to healthy, full term infants with the least complications.

**Nutritionally concentrated foods, rich in protein, and carbohydrates:**

**GRAINS:** brown rice, oats, cereals (oatmeal, granola, etc.), millet, corn, barley, bulgar, sprouted grains(including Brown rice breads, pastas, cereals, flour, etc.)

**LEGUMES:** green peas, lentils, chickpeas, alfalfa sprouts, mung beans, beans (kidney, lima, aduki, navy, soy and products made from them.)

**GREENS:** broccoli, collards, kale, kohlrabi, spinach, dark green lettuce, endive, romaine, beet and mustard greens, okra, zucchini squash, swiss chard, etc.

**Sprouted SEEDS:** sunflower seeds, sesame seeds, pumpkin seeds, flax etc. (sprouting reduces the fat content and increases the vitamin levels).

**Small amounts of NUTS:** almonds, cashews, walnuts, pecans, filberts, pistachios, macadamia, and nut butters (pour off the oil) from these.

**Vitamins** are an essential nutrient to the mother and child's' health. The cells of the body use active chemical substances called enzymes for protein production and metabolism. These enzymes need vitamins for their vital chemistry. There are two kind of vitamins, those that dissolve in water and those that dissolve in oil. **Water soluble vitamins** are not stored in the body and therefore must be consumed every day. These include Vitamin C, the B complex and Folic Acid. These vitamins are found in green, leafy vegetables, citrus fruits and nutritional yeast. The **oil soluble vitamins** are stored in the liver and include Vitamins A and E. They are found in yellow vegetables and melons, and in kale and broccoli.

**Minerals** such as potassium, sodium, selenium and iodine are needed for chemical and electrical reactions in the body. These are found in green leafy vegetables, grains, mushrooms, nutritional yeast and in sea vegetables (kombu, kelp, nori, dulse, etc.) Three more minerals are especially important to the pregnant woman: calcium, iron and zinc. Calcium is a vital element required for the healthy function of muscle, blood and bone in both mother and fetus. Green leafy vegetables, cabbage, legumes, corn tortillas, and seeds are particularly rich in calcium. Iron can be found also in green leafy vegetables, raisins, whole grains, seeds, legumes, hijiki seaweed, and dried fruits. Zinc is found in whole grains, green leafy vegetables, mushrooms, wheat germ, fortified cereals, tofu, miso, nuts and seeds.

However, some vitamins and minerals like Vitamin A, D, B-6 and iron, can have a toxic effect on mother and fetus if taken in excessive amounts. Check with your doctor to be sure your needs are being met with appropriate prenatal supplements.

**Water** is needed for blood flow, for the glands to secrete vital fluids and for the chemical reactions in the cells. The pregnant woman requires more fluid for making additional blood for herself, the baby and the amniotic fluid. Water, diluted fruit juices, vegetables juices and soups will help to supply the extra fluid needed.

## NURSING MOTHERS:

Breast-feeding is absolutely the best, most natural form of nutrition for your baby's health. The Healthy Aging plan provides nursing mothers with protein, vitamins, minerals, carbohydrates and fats needed for the rapid growth of the child in the first years of life. Nursing women who eat the conventional American diet consume meat, dairy products and fish that contain chemical contaminants such as hormones, pesticides and antibiotics. These substances pass through to the baby through the mothers breast milk.

Nursing or pregnant mothers who avoid allergy triggering foods (dairy milk, eggs, cheese, fish, nuts) may cut their babies risk of developing allergies by half according to a study from the June 19, 1992 Lancet. The babies were raised with significantly less asthma or eczema if the mothers followed an allergy free diet. Severe to mild allergies affect many races as they get older. This is only with cow or goat's milk; human milk would not cause a reaction. Unfortunately, human milk is not available at the store. However, even infants have been allergic to mother's milk if the mother is drinking cow's milk, which seems to pass on to the baby. The mother must stop drinking milk, according to Dr. Lendon Smith, pediatrician, and Dr. Paul Fliess, authorities on breast feeding.

The following guidelines for pregnant women will also meet the needs for lactating women. Be sure to eat iron and calcium rich foods, as the mother's stores may have been depleted during pregnancy. Water and a generous amount of fruits and vegetables are important to assure a large supply of breast milk. Be sure to monitor your weight and how you look. If you get too thin after being on this low-fat diet for several months eat more grains, rice, pasta, cereals, yams, and legumes. If you are too fatty, eat more soups, raw vegetable salads, fruit, and sprouts. In either case, avoid added proteins, fats, sugars, and salts. You and your children will be healthy and vital.

# Children & Teenagers

I'm sure you want to introduce your children to the proper way of eating. Here is an excellent guide for infant food introduction. At birth, you will want to start the child off with breast feeding. Breast milk is the best recommended food for the infant. You can breast feed the child to eighteen months and some children are breast fed until the age of two or a little longer. If for some reason, you cannot give the baby breast milk, you should contact La Leche League or some group that would help you to obtain breast milk. It is very important infants be breast fed to build up their immune system, to give proper nutrition and to avoid the danger of sudden infant death syndrome or crib death. If you must introduce a formula, a soy milk formula such as Isomil, Prosoybee or Similac would be safer than one based on cow's milk.

At six to seven months, you can introduce fresh fruits, such as bananas or peaches. Blend them so that the baby will enjoy them. Some basic baby foods available are good, just look for no added sugar or salt. At seven months, you can give the baby cooked green vegetables, sprouts and a little bit of avocado, along with a liquid vitamin. By the eight month you can introduce other cooked vegetables, yams, carrots and squash. At the tenth month the baby will thrive on starches, including potatoes, cereals and oats. At twelve months try wheat cereals and beans. Fourteen months introduce breads, pastas, and a small amount of almond butter. At this point, you can start feeding the baby the complex carbohydrate food that the family eats pureed from your meals.

The same diet that is good for you will be good for your baby. Don't get in the habit of feeding meat, dairy, eggs and fatty foods to your child just because you were raised on them. You'll never break the chain that way! You'll raise a baby that will have health problems, probably be overweight and not the opportunity that you have now following a good diet. Our children are precious to us and we must make the decision to adopt a healthy way of eating. If you start them on this plan from birth their taste buds will be adopted to proper nutrition.

I believe that most people eat sugar and fatty foods not so much because they like them, but because they become conditioned to eating them. A good example would be if you cut back on your salt consumption. If you then eat something with salt on it, it tastes too salty for your taste. Healthy eating started early helps to avoid poor nutrition habits later.

When your children approach their adolescent and teen years, they are obviously going to be exposed to the fatty, greasy foods. Don't worry if they occasionally eat these foods, because occasional use will not cause any harm. But, if they fall into a pattern of eating these high cholesterol, high fat foods regularly, then talk with your child about making better choices. Treat them like an adult and speak to them intelligently. They will respect you and if you find out what fruits and vegetables, grains, breads and so on that they like best, you can work around their diet. As the children are growing they need large amounts of grains, breads, pastas and rice for growth and energy. Give them smaller amounts of fruits and vegetables because they are lower in food density and calories.

These whole, natural foods also provide all the protein needed for a growing child. We have been brought up with the idea that dairy and meats are the high sources of protein. All foods have protein - potatoes, rice, corn and spaghetti are just a few examples of foods that are excellent sources of protein. Almost all foods have a natural source of fat, too. Unfortunately, we have all been conditioned to use excess sources of protein.

Ask your children what they like to eat. Make a thorough list - there may be some healthy foods you didn't know they do like! For example, your young child or teenagers list may include the following:

Nicholas **will eat**:
1. Old-fashioned oatmeal 2. Potatoes 3. Rice, Quick Brown 4. Bread
5. Tortillas 6. Beans - burritos 7. Oranges 8. Apples 9. Bananas
10. Grapes 11. Lettuce 12. Corn

Nicholas will **Avoid eating**:
1. Cheese 2. Milk 3. Meat 4. Chicken 5. Oils 6. candy

Weekly **REWARD** for good food choices: go to basketball game etc.

The above list comes from my son Nicholas, who was 6 years old at the time of this writing. He is not always perfect in adherence to this list. However, my son has a clear understanding of the purpose and the objective of good nutrition. I also supply Nicholas with additional motivation to stick to his diet by agreeing to play basketball with him. Also, I rent him his favorite video games when his compliance is particularly good. Generally, it's best to choose rewards that involve some kind of physical activity or outdoor outing the children enjoy.

Obviously, Cherish, Jason, and Lance have a different list of foods they like to eat, foods they must avoid, and rewards they want if they comply with a Healthy aging diet, supplements, and exercise plan. It's never too early to start your children on a health plan they will be able to follow for the rest of their lives. What a wonderful gift you are offering your children, the opportunity to prevent most all diseases, and live a long, healthy, happy life.

Don't ruin your children's motivation by sneaking in bad food and leaving it in the refrigerator. Food selection should be an example set by the parents. If you provide those nutritious foods in the cupboards and the refrigerator, your children will nibble on them instead of the greasy, fattening foods so prevalent today. Try having a pot of cooked brown rice, whole wheat spaghetti, salads or soups ready for your family to snack on during the day. You can make whole wheat pizza (NO CHEESE!) with mushrooms, tomatoes, bell peppers, pineapple or any other vegetables your children enjoy. You may need to motivate your children to eat properly by using some reward system. You might promise to go to a football game with them, or rent them a tape they want to see, etc.

Some people still worry about getting adequate vitamins and minerals in a high complex carbohydrate diet. These nutrients are easily obtained from plant foods, fortified foods and from supplements, without the need of any dairy or meat products. The following is a list of those nutrients that seem to cause the most misconception:

**Vitamin D:** This is necessary for calcium absorption, but is not really a "vitamin" at all. This is a hormone made by our bodies when sunlight falls on our skin. We only need 15 minutes a day of exposure to sunlight to meet our requirements.

**Vitamin B 12:** This vitamin is needed for healthy nerve function and is made only by bacteria. These bacteria, although found in animal foods, are also common soil organisms and are found on the surface of fresh vegetables. The body's need for this vitamin is very small - .5 millionths of a gram for infants to 3 millionths of a gram at 7 years of age. It is unlikely any child eating a balanced diet to be deficient in B-12. However, because B-12 deficiency is serious and completely preventable, you can supplement with any of the following: use sublingual drops or spray, or Crush a few 25-microgram tablets of B-12 and add a pinch of this powder to the baby's cooked food several times per week. Give the child a vitamin supplement that contains B-12. It is best to begin B-12 supplements when the baby is six months old.

**Zinc:** This mineral is necessary for a strong immune system. It is found in fortified cereals, sprouted whole grains, leafy greens, nuts and wheat germ.

**Iron:** Iron is vital to keep pace with a child's production of new blood. Iron rich foods such as greens, legumes, raisins, dates, apricots, iron-enriched cereals and breads should meet your child's needs. Test your child's blood once a year for anemia. If necessary, you can then add more iron-containing foods or iron supplements.

**Calcium:** This mineral is found in seeds, greens, nuts, legumes, tofu and drinking water. A child following the Healthy Aging diet should have no difficulty meeting the required 200 to 800 milligrams daily. If there is any question of consuming adequate calcium in the diet, liquid calcium supplements or calcium-fortified soy-milk can be used.

**Motivating your children** to eat properly, you are giving them an important gift - the gift of health and happiness. Spend time educating your children. Most parents allow the **TV to baby-sit** for up to 4 or more hours per day, seven days a week. The average child sees more than 20,000 commercials a year, and by the age of 21, over one million commercials! Children tend to believe commercials and need to be taught the difference and the truth. Nine out of ten ads on Saturday morning TV are for greasy, fatty, high cholesterol, sugar loaded junk food. Children's programming contains an average of 26 violent acts per hour, while prime time has five acts of violence. Teens see over 100,000 ads for alcohol before drinking age. Advertisers spend over $800,000 million a year on ads aimed at kids. Children under 12 and teenagers influence their parents to spend over $160 billion a year. Watch TV with your children and talk about the misleading advertising. You may be able to extend the quality of their lives and of their offspring in coming generations. Won't you help reduce the rate of obesity, heart disease and cancer in children by getting to the cause of the problem?

# XV

∞

# Save Your Life Reduce Your Cholesterol Level

---

Your cholesterol level will not affect your weight or your energy level; however, it is a problem that has been tragically overlooked for many years. Cholesterol and atherosclerosis are major problems in America and the overall degree of this problem is not fully understood by our society. We know the death rate from heart disease has decreased slightly, However, it still affects millions of Americans.

Consider the fact strokes are the second leading cause of death. Then combine heart attacks and the number of people who die of strokes and we have diseases that kill more than 50% of all Americans. The pain and the suffering these diseases cause our country is tragic and yet, we continue to ignore dietary treatment. As Americans, it is important that we have the information available to us about the low fat, zero cholesterol Healthy Aging Plan.

Several years ago I worked with stroke victims in physical therapy in the critical care units. These people had lives just like you and I. They had families. They led happy and successful lives. Then, one unexpected day they had a stroke. Overnight their whole world crumbled and they became bedridden and in need of constant care.

Stroke rehabilitation is a laborious, slow process. It may take six months before a stroke victim can actually walk on their own, and even then many victims never regain full function. Half their body is paralyzed simply because arteries leading to the brain became severely clogged with cholesterol. Consequently, part of the brain dies due to lack of oxygen. Some stroke victims can no longer speak clearly, if that part of the brain was affected. Think about it - the brain never stops working. When you go to sleep, your brain is still functioning and coordinating your whole body.

Circulation to your brain will also effect performance, mental clarity, and your energy level. Have a carotid artery ultrasound (ask the doctor or technician to identify for you even the smallest of cholesterol atherosclerotic plaques). Ask your doctor to refer you for a noninvasive, Ultra Fast CT Scan of the heart. The doctors were amazed to find how clean my arteries were without any calcification or cholesterol! When I was asked how I did it? I responded. "The Healthy Aging program works...try it!"

These are very serious problems: cholesterol, heart disease and strokes. There is a tendency for Americans to ignore something they cannot see. I have conducted over 3,000 seminars in the last 20 years and I spent most of the seminar time educating people about the importance of cholesterol control. When a patient comes to the seminar overweight, fatigued and lacking energy, they immediately know what they want. They want to lose weight and increase their energy. Since we have a solution for them, these people are easy to work with because they will follow the guidelines for losing weight and increasing energy. However, the people with high cholesterol levels don't believe it's a problem.

Cholesterol is the silent killer. Since there are no nerve endings in the arteries, you don't know cholesterol is building up. Unfortunately a massive heart attack or stroke is the first symptom some people will experience. Then you'll seek treatment, but at that point, there is already irreversible damage.

Special interest groups such as the meat, egg and dairy industries are trying to divert attention from their high cholesterol foods by placing the blame on saturated fats. They tell you that the Eskimos and the Masai tribe in Africa eat a high cholesterol diet and are free of heart disease. Yet in *Scientific American, September, 1971* in was found Eskimos living in the central arctic region eat less than 23% fat have no heart disease, while the coastal Eskimos eating blubber fat have a high incidence of stroke. The Masai tribe according to Dr. Mann, eat blood of cows and sour milk, and they pass treadmill tests because they're in great shape from herding cattle over 20 miles a day. However on autopsy, they have massive plaques in their arteries. These groups claim palm oil and coconut oil, which are high in saturated fat, are the cause of elevated cholesterol levels. People are now buying vegetable oils high in monounsaturated and polyunsaturated fats mistakenly believing these are better for them.

In the *Journal of American Medical Association, March 23, 1990, Vol. 263,* Dr. David Blankenhorn of U.S.C. reported his studies on the effects of fats and the development of atherosclerotic lesions in human coronary arteries. The results shocked the margarine and oil industry since it was proven all fats including polyunsaturated, monounsaturated, saturated and fatty acids (lauric, oleic and linoleic acids) more than 26% of calories from fat caused cholesterol lesions in the heart arteries in less than two years. Those people who were protected from cholesterol lesions ate the least amount of all types of fats.

The public is also misled by believing if they avoid saturated fats they can continue to eat their high cholesterol foods. I can't tell you how many people who come to the seminars still eat at least one or two eggs a week, and think it's safe for them. Of course, we know eggs are one of the most potent sources of cholesterol. You should never eat more than one or two eggs per year. That would be only if you were unaware they were in a recipe, such as a bakery item.

I believe part of the reason people continue to eat high cholesterol foods comes from watching television and the brain-washing that conditions them.

A study showed that the average person during their lifetime spends:
Speaking with their **child** (two weeks or 30 sec per day), **Brushing** their teeth(3 weeks), Conversing with **spouse** (100 days or 4 min per day), Sitting at **red lights**(150 days), Opening **junk mail** (200 days), Searching for things they **lost**(one year), **Exercising** (two years, if they exercise one-half hour a day), Attending **meetings**(three years), **Cleaning** their house(four years), **Waiting** in lines(five years), **Eating**(six years), In the **bathroom** (seven years), and the big time waster is **Watching television**(over **23 years** -ASTONISHING!)

The dairy and meat industries promote their products and bombard us with **advertising**. The average child will watch over **100,000 commercials** by the time they're a teenager. These commercials claim eggs, meat and cheese build strong bodies and "milk has something for every body." Commercials about beer, Pepsi, Coke and candy will complete the child's' nutritional education. Spokespersons paid by these special interest groups mislead the public into believing they can eat as much meat, eggs, and cheese as they wish. Deliberately eating these products ignores the fact cholesterol kills more people in America than any other cause of death.

Dr. Wong and Dr. Gold reported the results of their study on over 1,000 youngsters age two to age 20 (November 1990 *American Heart Association* Meeting). They found over 53 % of children with a dangerously high cholesterol level, 200 mg/dl or higher, watch television two or more hours per day. Those who watched four or more hours per day were four times as likely to have high cholesterol levels.

Cholesterol building up in the arteries is a leading cause of senility. By the age of 60, many senior citizens in our country are completely senile and end up in nursing homes needing constant care. If we look at the issues, we know that cholesterol is the culprit. Even a two-year-old who is fed high cholesterol foods can develop a build-up. By the time he is three, he'll already have fatty streaks in his arteries. That is how early it starts.

In Finland they have the highest cholesterol level in the world and the highest death rate from heart attack and stroke. Their infants are born with a higher cholesterol level than the worldwide averages because the mothers are eating a very high cholesterol diet. In this country our teenagers eat a high cholesterol diet of cheeseburgers, fried foods, beef burritos with added cheese. With all this cholesterol, it's inevitable that a teenager will develop clogged arteries. When they reach 30 or 40 years old, the first heart attacks appear. Every day 3,425 people across the country have a heart attack (1,250,000 per year), and over half these people will die immediately. Heart attacks occur in teenagers, but we don't hear much about them because they're not as frequent as in a 40-year-old. So, we have to start this nutritional plan of zero cholesterol and low fat intake.

Add **soluble fiber**(soluble means it absorbs fluid) to your diet. An experiment using *Gum Arabic*, a natural soluble fiber that absorbs bile in the digestive tract. Bile is made up principally of cholesterol, and soluble fiber adheres to cholesterol and fat and increases excretion of LDL cholesterol by 21% and triglycerides by 30%. This can increase chance of survival from clogged arteries. Over 90% of Americans do not get enough fiber in there diet. Be sure to add products rich in soluble fiber such as *pysllium husk* from the sunflower seed family, apple *pectin*, citrus pectin, *Oat bran, Nopal* from cactus to reduce fat and *Glucomannan* (Konjac Root powder).

In the last ten years there has been a significant decrease in the number of deaths from atherosclerosis (cholesterol plaques in the arteries). One study estimated that over 180,000 people are alive today in the U.S. because they learned how to lower and keep their cholesterol level down. Stop Smoking campaigns has also helped to decrease the death rate. However, the number one causes of death in the U.S. are still heart disease, stroke and cancer.

**Degenerative-Diseases:... 1994-to-1996**
**(Most recent year for complete statistics)**
**TOTAL COST OVER ONE TRILLION DOLLARS!**

| | |
|---|---|
| Heart Disease & Hypertension | 738,000 deaths / 60 million afflicted |
| Stroke | 154,000 deaths / 3,890,000 disabled |
| Cancer cost $104 billion | 480,000 deaths /1,360,000 new cases |
| Accidents | 92,000 deaths |
| Obstructing lung disease | 78,000 deaths |
| Pneumonia ~ Flu | 68,600 deaths |
| Diabetes | 37,800 deaths |
| Suicide | 29,600 deaths |
| Cirrhosis of Liver | 26,000 deaths |
| Atherosclerosis | 23,100 deaths |
| AIDS - drug related abuse | 4,400 deaths |

At Healthy aging clinics, we are often asked What is the difference between fat and cholesterol? **Fat** provides calories; yet, in excess it is the major contributor to obesity and to many diseases that affects our culture. A high fat diet of oils, margarine, whole milk, cheese, meat, etc. can increase the levels of fat in your blood (**triglycerides**) which along with other causes leads to the risk of:

High *Triglyceride* causes:

1. **HIGH BLOOD PRESSURE** (blood thickened by fat)
2. **ARTHRITIS** (low oxygen from fat causing destruction of joints)
3. **DIABETES** (fat desensitizing insulin causing elevated glucose)
4. **BREAST** and **COLON CANCER** (fat causing excessive production of cancer causing hormones and chemicals)
5. **CHRONIC FATIGUE** (high fat levels in the blood, reduces the oxygen carrying capacity of red blood cells to the brain)
6. **GLAUCOMA** (fat increases cortisone levels in the eyes causing swelling, restriction of fluid flow that can result in damage to the retinal nerves of the eye and blindness)
7. **MULTIPLE SCLEROSIS** (fat damages the nerves of the body from reduced oxygen carrying capacity of the blood)
8. **ATHEROSCLEROSIS** (low oxygen levels caused by fat forces more cholesterol deposits into the arteries)

In comparison, **cholesterol** is much different from fat. First because Cholesterol cannot cause you to gain weight since it lacks calories. Unlike fat, you can't see cholesterol in food, since it's permeated equally throughout all animal tissue. This is why there is just as much cholesterol in the white part of chicken or fish as there is in the skin or fat portions. **HIGH CHOLESTEROL** levels can lead to:

1. **ATHEROSCLEROSIS** -narrowing of arteries and capillaries.
2. **HEART ATTACK** from cholesterol blocked heart arteries
3. **STROKE** -clogged and weakened arteries to the brain.
4. **SENILITY** -loss of brain function due to clogged arteries.
5. **IMPOTENCY**-unable to achieve erection, because cholesterol narrows arteries to the penis.
6. **PROSTATE CANCER** (cholesterol build up in the prostate gland restricts oxygen to the gland inducing mutated cancerous cells).
7. **CATARACTS**-lens of eye fills with cholesterol causing blindness.
8. **GANGRENE** (restricted blood flow to the extremities: fingers, toes, hands and feet, leading to numbness, tissue death & amputation caused by cholesterol build up).
9. **KIDNEY FAILURE** (clogged arteries to the kidneys).

**Supplements to help with the reduction of cholesterol: Alfalfa**, Aloe Vera, Cayenne, DHEA, Growth Hormone, Devils Claw, Garlic, Parsley, Capsicum, Lecithin, Licorice, Melatonin, Suma, Vitamin E, papaya, chromium, L-Cartinine, Kelp, yellow dock, psyllium husk, Vitamin C, Vitamin B Complex, milk thistle, grapefruit pectin, grape seed, rutin, guar, hibiscus, black walnut, chickweed, cinnamon cloves, dandelion, echinacea, false unicorn, fenugreek, pumpkin and Cholesterad®.

**Stroke, brain & spinal cord injury** can improve if hyperbaric oxygen therapy is begun immediately. Portable home units are now available. Hyperbaric Oxygen Therapy (HBOT) has been written about in over 30,000 scientific studies published in medical and clinical journals. HBOT chamber forces extra oxygen into the body under pressure, oxygen dissolves into all of the body's fluids, including the plasma, the lymph, the cerebrospinal fluid surrounding the brain and spinal cord. These fluids can carry extra oxygen by seeping to areas where circulation is poor or blocked, promote new capillaries, new connective tissue, and enhance white blood cells ability to fight infectious bacteria, viruses, fungi, and parasites.

Forty-six medical schools in the U.S. and virtual all Italian medical schools, Chinese and Russian hospitals (3,000 chambers) use or teach hyperbaric medicine. Unfortunately, there are less than 400 Oxygen chambers being used in the U.S., treating only 100,000 patients a year. There is no *patent* on oxygen therapy, so educating doctors and health care professionals has been slow.

I believe the new portable Hyperbaric chamber (less than $16,000 unit) made by **Hyper-Oxy** is the solution to wide scale use. These Durable home treatment units are now available which weigh less than 30 pounds and fit in a carry bag. A compressor pumps purified air to maintain pressure, while special valves assure constant air exchange and prevent buildup of carbon dioxide inside the chamber. An oxygen mask placed in the chamber allows breathing of oxygen under pressure. Hospitals and home care patients will be able to accelerate healing after surgery by 30%, save lives, suffering and reduce health care costs.

Each year, Americans suffer over 25 million emergency room visits for serious **accidents, burns, wounds, headaches, hearing loss, head** and **spinal cord injuries** (car, violence etc.). Also, 800,000 people are **poisoned** from household chemicals or carbon monoxide fumes. **Stroke victims** (third most frequent cause of death and a leading cause of disability) require immediate therapy and long term help. SPECT scans of the brain show rapid recovery from stroke when provided hyperbaric oxygen therapy within hours of a stroke. **Peripheral vascular disease** can cause pain and spasms in limbs, feet, or hands and is responsible for more than 6 million lost workdays per year in the U.S. Studies show a 40% improvement after HBOT. **Multiple Sclerosis** patients improve in 70% of the cases from HBOT according to the *New England Journal of Medicine, Jan 1983.*

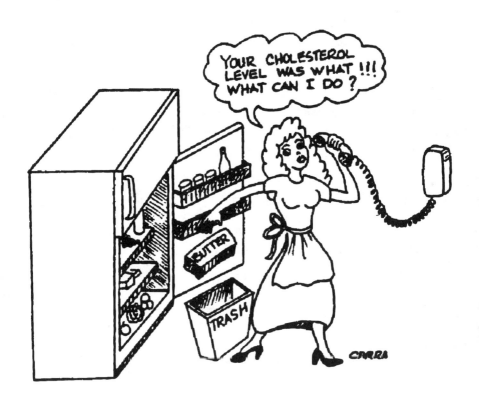

# XVI

# Blood Pressure & Hypertension

Over fifty million Americans have high blood pressure (also known as hypertension) and it threatens the lives of one out of every four adults and children. That message doesn't always reach receptive ears, especially when most doctors and patients depend on drugs to cover up symptoms instead of using diet and exercise to treat the cause.

One of the main concerns is most people who have high blood pressure will not seek treatment. Many people never even know they have high blood pressure. Why? Because there are no symptoms and it doesn't hurt. You really don't know you have high blood pressure until a doctor or health professional examines your pressure.

Think of high blood pressure as a disease that involves the whole body, not just as something that has gone wrong with the pressure. If your blood pressure is higher, such as 140/90, then we become very concerned. If you maintain a high blood pressure level over ten or twenty years, the arteries begin to become affected. It accelerates deterioration of your arteries, which can leave you susceptible to arterial blowout, possibly a stroke or an aneurysm.

Of course, these can all be very dangerous. Dr. Albert Einstein had an abdominal aneurysm and every time his heart would beat, the weakened point in the artery lining would bulge out. Just as on a basketball, if there is a weakened point, a bubble will form. Unfortunately, one day that abdominal aneurysm burst and Dr. Einstein died. Another problem with high blood pressure is it affects the main target organs: the brain, kidneys and possibly the liver. These organs can become damaged from continual high pressure.

Another name for high blood pressure is hypertension. Some people mistakenly believe high blood pressure is due to tension or being upset. The reality is high blood pressure is related to the thickness of the blood (fat thickens blood), or the total volume of blood (salt ratio higher than potassium retains fluid increasing volume) and the elasticity of the artery wall (cholesterol plaque hardens the artery). A normal blood pressure is usually 110/70, the measure of pressure exerted on the artery lining. When your heart beats, the blood going from the heart through the arteries can exert 110 millimeters of mercury of pressure. Between beats there is a pressure (70 mm) exerted by the arteries to return the blood to the heart. We have found lower blood pressure, 110/70 or 100/60, is now considered better than 120/80. The chances of heart attacks are double at a diastolic pressure over 80.

If we examine various cultures throughout the world, we find groups of people who eat large amounts of **salt** have an alarming rate of high blood pressure. For example, 40% of the population in northern Japan eat from 18 to 30 grams of salt daily, have high blood pressure and one of the highest death rates from stroke (arterial blowout) in the world. If we compare this Japanese culture to the New Guinea natives who eat a low-salt diet and low-fat diet, we find they have no incidence of high blood pressure, and even when they reach age 60, they still have a 110/60 blood pressure.

What is it about salt that increases the blood pressure? Salt causes fluid retention. If you use salt in your foods, this excess salt will absorb fluid into your bloodstream, adding 5-7 extra pounds of water weight to your bloodstream. This extra weight will create more pressure every time your heart beats. For example, when you turn on the garden hose and force more fluid through it, the pressure goes up.

We know high blood pressure is **not hereditary**. Studies were done on Japanese who migrated to other countries where they eat less salt, and their blood pressure began to drop down. In another study of high school students in Japan, one group was taught how to lower salt in the diet. Another group, the control group, continued eating as much salt as they wanted. At the end of the study, the group who ate the most salt had somewhat higher blood pressure. The group who kept their salt intake down maintained a normal blood pressure.

In a 1975 study, Dr. Iacono of the Agricultural Department instructed a group of people who were eating 10 grams of salt per day (the average American intake) to continue eating the same amount of salt while cutting back on the amount of **fat** in their diet. Instead of eating the usual 35-43% fat diet, he showed them how to reduce their fat intake to under 25% fat. They switched to nonfat milk instead of whole milk, chicken, fish and turkey instead of red, fatty meats. They cut back on the use of butter, margarine and oils, and started steaming and broiling their foods.

Within ten days, these patients lowered their blood pressure a full 10%, both the systolic and diastolic numbers. When they started eating the same **high fat diet** as before, their blood pressure rose. Dr. Iacono had discovered the amount of fat in the diet affected blood pressure far more than the amount of salt.

Don't misunderstand - we're suggesting you do reduce the salt in your diet, but once you reduce the salt, the far greater cause of high blood pressure is fat in the diet.

April 17, 1997, in *The New England Journal of Medicine,* using a low-fat diet rich in fruits, vegetables, and nonfat products, "blood pressure lowered as much as any single drug treatment, and did it in only two weeks!" This study using Dietary Approaches to Stop Hypertension (DASH) according to Suzanne Oparil, cardiologist and a past president of the American Heart Association said "the most dramatic effect of diet on blood pressure I've ever seen-as good as or better than (the effect of) many drugs." The study cost over $7 million dollars and was sponsored by the National Heart, Lung, and Blood Institute, on 459 adults with hypertension defined as above 140/ 90 to 160/100. The most successful group in the study consumed **over 10 servings of fruits and vegetables** a day combined with nonfat or low in saturated fat products. Sound familiar, doesn't it, like the Healthy Aging Plan? The diet highest in vegetables and fruit lowered the blood pressure by more than double compared to less than 8.5 servings of fruits and vegetables a day during the 8 week study. The people with the highest blood pressures reduced the most. "Everybody in the study had the same sodium intake" from salt, and "we didn't allow folks to lose or gain weight." They didn't want people to say the results came from weight loss or less salt intake.

If you reduce salt in the diet and your blood pressure doesn't come down to normal, you have to search for other possible causes. If a doctor examines you, and cannot find the problem, you may be told you have "essential hypertension," which means "of unknown cause." At this point, you may be given medications to control your blood pressure.

But, **medications** are no longer considered a safe form of treatment. 35% of those on these medications must stop taking them because of serious side effects. *Diuretics* may double your chances of sudden death due to **heart failure**. These drugs raise your blood **cholesterol, triglycerides** and **glucose.** Sir William Osler, a famous physician, stated, "One of the first duties of the physician is to educate the masses not to take medicine." Benjamin Franklin said, "It is the best physician that knows the worthlessness of most medicines." If you are on medications now, there is a safer, more effective solution.

If you follow our natural approach to lowering blood pressure, you'll be much safer than depending on medications for the rest of your life. *Prolonged use* of these **medications** can cause **kidney damage** and high urea nitrogen levels, which can cause **kidney failure.** You may develop **gouty arthritis** because uric acid levels elevate from certain blood pressure medications. These drugs also can cause elevation of the blood glucose level and you could become **diabetic.** Surprisingly, as stated earlier in this book, **male impotency** can result as a side effect from blood pressure medications.

Research studies showed over 50% of the men tested became sexually impotent because the blood flow was reduced so much from the blood pressure medications they were unable to maintain an erection. These drugs have also reported to cause apathy and diminished sexual excitability. Beta-blocker drugs used to lower blood pressure alter brain function. Side effects include reports of failing memory, headaches, dizziness, drowsiness, depression, nightmares and a decline in intellectual power.

According to Dr. Cleaves Bennett, M.D., hypertension specialist, there are four major types of medication that are currently used in the treatment of high blood pressure: the diuretics, the blockers, the vasodilators and the inhibitors.

1) The best the **diuretics** can do is rid your body of some salt. You could do that by cutting down on the amount of salt you eat, while increasing the use of potassium rich foods like watermelon, carrots, tomatoes, apples and sprouts.

Diuretics often don't work if they're not used correctly and if they don't work it is harder for the other drugs to work as well. A good diet would do what diuretics do - and do it better.

2) The **blockers** leave you drowsy when they work, and when they don't make you drowsy, they can't control your blood pressure in a routine domestic crisis or a traffic jam. According to the *British Medical Journal, March 7, 1998(316:741)* the use of calcium channel blockers, increased the rate of suicide by five times compared to nonusers. This drug causes severe depression, yet it's annual sales are over $8 billion dollars. In the *New England Journal of Medicine* January 8, 1998, found that 96% of the doctors in favor of using these harmful drugs had financial ties with the pharmaceutical manufactures. Stress management and diet would do what the blockers do much better.

3) The **vasodilators** diminish the pressure in the blood vessels by acting directly on the muscles of the arterioles. A low-fat diet, rich in potassium from vegetables, fruit and salt reduction would do a better job of controlling the fluid content of the blood vessels, and stress management with exercise would relax the muscles in the arterioles more effectively.

4) The **endocrine inhibitors**: Captopril is a drug that blocks the formation of angiotensin, a hormone that can raise the blood pressure profoundly. This overactive renin-angiotensin problem rarely occurs. However, when it does it is usually caused by cholesterol blockages of the arteries leading to the kidneys. The drug Captopril only works for a while, until the body learns to counteract the effect of the drug by making more of the hormone.

The best solution is to unclog the arteries to the kidneys by the Healthy Aging Diet. It may take two or three years, but diet does get to the cause of the problem instead of covering it up with drugs.

Many patients assume the medications they take must be good for them because their blood pressure is lower. It simply isn't true. *The Journal of the American Medical Association* published a recent report entitled, "Multiple Risk Factor Intervention Trial (1982). The authors described their results as "ambiguous but disquieting." They found the use of pharmacologic therapy - drugs-in the treatment of some hypertensives seems associated with "an increased **coronary heart disease** mortality." In simple English, they found that taking a diuretic for high blood pressure might lower the blood pressure while raising the total risk of dying from heart disease.

Unfortunately, most doctors can't possibly read all the articles in all the medical journals. A study published in the *American Journal of Medicine (1982)* showed many doctors are more influenced by the glossy color handouts drug salesmen pass around than they are by articles in the medical journals. Drug companies make their advertising literature much easier to read than the journals, with their small print and extensive footnotes.

As a result, research that encourages the use of drugs is often more familiar to doctors. After all, no one goes from doctor to doctor promoting wellness plans, because if you take care of yourself through diet and exercise, you may not need any drugs. That approach won't sell anything. I assure you that for every drug there are a company representative knocking on the doctors' doors showing beautiful brochures with data to support the drugs' use. If the representative can sell your doctor on a drug, then the doctor can sell hundreds of patients on it and there are huge profits to be made.

The first week you start our program, you should see your doctor. Under a doctor's supervision, you will need to decrease slowly, day by day, the drug dosage you're taking now and monitor your blood pressure. Generally, you should begin reducing or stopping the strongest first, the one that causes the worst side effects. Usually, the strongest medications are the ones a doctor adds last. Proceed under your doctor's supervision, while monitoring your blood pressure in the doctor's office and at home. Begin with the most powerful drugs. When the dosage is large, your doctor may begin by cutting the amount of one type of medications by a third or half as a first step. Wait about three days before beginning the next decrease in dosage of this medication. When you have reached the smallest dosage in which the medication is packaged, then the next step is to stop it altogether.

If with the dietary change, blood pressure falls to levels that are too low to be on medications, such as 110/70 or lower, or if a person becomes dizzy, then the dosages should be lowered more rapidly. When adjusting medications in this manner, try to keep the blood pressure below 160/100. Don't worry if the pressure is this high for a few days. This elevation for a short time does not place you in any extra danger.

However, most people with high blood pressure have a very serious disease of the arteries and therefore are at a high risk of having a hazardous complication. Even so, if a stroke or heart attack did occur while an individual was making adjustments, often it would be a coincidence. The actual cause of these events would be many years of serious damage to the arteries from abuses caused by diet and lifestyle, not from the reduction in medication and the slight rise in blood pressure, which sometimes follows a lower dosage.

Actually, during this short period of adjustment, the danger is greater from too much medication than too little. Over- enthusiastic treatment of blood pressure can be dangerous. The attempt to lower blood pressure to normal levels with medication in-patients with extensive atherosclerosis has been shown to result in a fivefold increase in heart attacks.

Beta-blockers should be reduced slowly, because rapid withdrawal can cause bothersome strong or rapid heartbeats. There is also some evidence that too rapid a decrease in dosage of beta-blockers will cause chest pains and heart attacks in susceptible patients. On the other hand, withdrawal of some medications, such as clonidine, may cause a rapid rise in blood pressure, with symptoms of nervousness, agitation and headache. The medication should be reduced slowly, at intervals of three days.

Your goal is to lower your blood pressure to 110/70 or less without medication. Some people will not reach this ideal pressure, even following a strict low-salt, low-fat vegetarian diet and clean lifestyle, because the damage to the circulatory system is already too severe. Also, small minorities of people have hypertension from causes other than years of poor diet and lifestyle practices, which need attention in addition to changes in their habits. A doctor will need to identify these rare cases.

If we examine people on a high fat diet and look at their bloodstream, the red blood cells are stuck together. Fat, whether animal or vegetable in origin, will cause the blood cells to stick together and thicken the blood. This forces the blood pressure to go up, because the cells can barely get through the smaller blood vessels, the capillaries. When you start on the Healthy Aging Plan reducing fat and exercise 30 minutes or more per day, the red blood cells become evenly separated rapidly. Your blood pressure will start to come down almost immediately.

I'd like to summarize the best ways to lower blood pressure. The first and most important step is to reduce fat in your diet and start eating more water rich complex carbohydrates (ten or more servings a day of sprouts, vegetables and fruit). The second would be to cut back on your salt use. Instead of salt on your foods and in cooking, use onion powder, garlic powder, cayenne pepper and other spices. Step three is losing weight. If you're overweight, the body has to work harder to maintain blood flow.

Another way to lower blood pressure is through aerobic exercise, such as brisk walking, jogging or using mini-trampolines. We have found aerobic exercising for one-half to an hour per day, will help to reduce the fat levels in your bloodstream and dilate blood vessels. Studies show for most people, blood pressure will come down dramatically within seven weeks. Recent studies show caffeine in soda drinks or coffee, nicotine in cigarettes, and alcohol will promote high blood pressure.

We have also found reducing cholesterol intake in the diet may help to reduce blood pressure significantly. **Cholesterol reduction** is important because if your arteries are loaded with plaques, it will be more difficult for the blood to flow through the clogged arteries. Reducing cholesterol then, is one of your goals, and it also can help to prevent aneurysms and the weakening of the artery linings.

Reduction of stress is also important, although continued stress is not the main cause of high blood pressure. It may temporarily elevate your blood pressure while you're upset, but stress cannot maintain it chronically day after day, year after year. If your blood pressure is elevated, you need to improve the blood flow first and then start working toward reducing stress.

You'll need to see your doctor to reduce medications as needed. When you start following these points, you're blood pressure will come down rapidly, almost dramatically. If you do not reduce blood pressure medications within two to four weeks, you may have too low of a blood pressure because our plan is so powerful! One possible symptom of too low blood pressure would be to become weak or dizzy when you try to get up after sitting.

With our health plan we have one of the highest success rates in the country helping people to control blood pressure. Dr. Jeremiah Stamler, cardiologist at Northwestern University Medical School stated in *Science,*

April 18, 1997, after reviewing the *DASH study* rich in vegetables and fruit, low in saturated animal fat, "we have the potential for applying the knowledge learned here to markedly blunt the rise of blood pressure with age."...using a Healthy Aging diet! Add this with daily exercise, hormones, herbs, vitamins, minerals and enzymes.

**Herbs, hormones, vitamins and minerals to lower blood pressure**
To lower blood pressure be sure to include: homeopathic human growth hormone, IGF-1, DHEA, progesterone, testosterone, CoQ10, Una de Gato, Bee Pollen, garlic, white willow, hawthorn, maidenhair, L-Carnitine, potassium, magnesium, Vitamin B12, niacin, zinc, citrus bioflavonoids, rutin, hawthorn berries, capsicum, peppermint, and ginger. To strengthen the artery walls, take major and trace minerals as 92 ionic minerals (ionic is 1,000 times smaller than colloidal or chelated minerals to enhance absorption into the cells), and phyto Veggie & PhytoOrchard capsules (blend of juices from organic vegetables and fruit).

**STRESS**
A problem that we all face in our fast-paced society is stress. Stress does not directly cause high blood pressure. For example, you're upset, you have a fight with a loved one - spouse, boyfriend, girlfriend, etc. and what happens? Perhaps you neglect yourself, you don't exercise or you eat all the wrong foods. You might get the nervous nibbles and start eating compulsively. Stress has a very powerful effect on our lives and how we live. I'd like to share with you ways to reduce stress and get control of your life.

Are you a Type A personality? Are you under a great deal of stress? For instance, do you rush your speech? Do you hurry other people's speech? Do you hurry when you eat? Do you never seem to catch up? Do you schedule more activities than you have time to complete? Do you often try to do several things at once? Notice how often you'll be driving on the freeway and see other drivers shaving, drinking coffee and reading at the same time!

Do you drive fast most of the time? Most of us are in such a hurry, instead of scheduling enough time to get to our destination. This can be very upsetting, especially when you become impatient if others are driving too slowly. Do you have an intense drive, a constant struggle to get ahead? Do you detest wasting time and race with the clock, constantly looking at your watch? Of course, having an intense drive, struggling to get ahead and watching your time is all part of an executive's lifestyle. However, you can still be in control without the damaging effects of stress.

Do you have little time for relaxation, intimacy or enjoying your environment? In other words, do you set aside time to go to the movies, the beach, admire a sunset? You need to schedule time for activities you really enjoy. Some people have a difficult time thinking of things that they like to do. Do you compete with others to get ahead and have trouble returning to normal after intense stress? These are some important areas to consider because if stress is affecting your health and the way you function, then you have a major problem.

When we are under stress, we all react the same way with what we call the "fight or flight" syndrome. Your brain will immediately relay a signal and release certain hormones, including ACTH and adrenaline, if you become upset or perceive stress. These hormones enter the bloodstream and cause rapid physiological changes. You breathe faster, your heart beats faster, your blood sugar levels increase and the digestive tract slows down. The muscles in your hands and feet tighten up. Your hands get cold because your blood vessels are constricting. Your blood pressure goes up while you're under stress, your eyes dilate and your hair stands on end.

In primitive times this type of reaction was to your benefit. If you had to run or fight to save your life, you could meet the demands with this excess intensity, energy and concentration. But, let's imagine you're driving on the freeway and someone cuts in front of you. You grab the steering wheel, you honk the horn and you yell at the other driver. You get so upset and you go through those stress responses. Several hours later, the bloodstream is fired up with adrenaline and this can cause you considerable problems.

Stress can cause an increase in stomach acids that are secreted in the abdominal area. If there is no fibrous food present in the stomach, the acids begin to eat away at the stomach lining, which is the principal cause of ulcers. We have also found stress-related ulcers can be reduced significantly if we stay in control of the situation.

To protect yourself from ulcers, you must also follow a high fiber protective diet. A bland diet, devoid of fiber, in the past was the recommended plan to follow if you had ulcers. We now know that diets lacking fiber will increase the development rate of ulcers.

In a study conducted during World War II, groups of officers, safe behind enemy lines, were examined and found to have a high rate of ulcers. These men were eating processed foods, white bread, eggs, butter, cheese, etc., all foods containing no fiber. This was very surprising because the men on the front lines who were shot at, in a life threatening situation and who were under a great deal more stress, had no ulcers. Why? The men on the front lines were only served basic staples - whole oatmeal, whole brown rice, whole wheat bread, potatoes, etc. They had none of the processed, sugary, salty foods available only to the officers.

Based on this evidence, a **high fiber diet** will help to reduce the ulcer significantly, usually within a period of two years. To increase your fiber intake, eat beans, peas, yams, raw carrots and prunes. All of these foods are rich in soothing fiber. You can use additional wheat bran in your whole grain cereals. Eat large amounts of brown rice and whole oatmeal.

What is it about fiber that protects you from ulcers? We have found eating frequent meals (5-10 meals daily) of high fiber, complex carbohydrate food creates artificial mucus lining in the intestinal tract and in the stomach. Even if the stomach's acids are secreted when you become upset, the artificial mucus lining will protect the stomach lining from being eaten away. This prevents ulcers and bleeding ulcers.

We want to help you reduce stress directly. One of the most effective techniques is called the "Quieting Response." Dr. Charles Strobel, using biofeedback equipment developed this technique. When Dr. Strobel noticed people upset, he'd hook them up to his equipment and teach them how to calm and relax themselves by listening to the machine and monitoring their progress through biofeedback. Although the equipment was effective, he found it was difficult for people to transfer what they had learned from these machines to their day-to-day environment. Because of this problem, Dr. Strobel developed this very effective technique called the "Quieting Response." You can use it any time during the day, as often as needed, whenever you are under stress.

Here are the steps to the "Quieting Response." First, when you recognize you're under stress, you need to smile immediately. You may not know it, but you can create 250,000 different facial expressions and the smile nuerologically effects the brain and begins to calm you. Earlier, you learned the brain is the first to perceive stress and releases these hormones, so when you smile, you're beginning to gain control. Of course, if you are in an intense situation, such as an argument, and you smile outwardly, you may get punched in the nose! In that situation, it would obviously be better to smile inwardly. It may take a little practice, but it works very well.

The next step is to say to yourself, "I am in control and calm and I can handle this situation." This is very important to keep repeating to yourself.

The third step is to take two slow, easy, deep breaths through your nose. Relax and breathe. Remember that this is all happening in less than six seconds, so you need to create it as an automatic response.

Then, you need to be sure your jaw is loose and relaxed, because if your jaw is tight, it's going to cause stress. Your tongue should be resting on the lower part of your jaw, and your shoulders should be limp and relaxed. Be in control of your body and your mind. Keep repeating to yourself "I am in control."

The final step is to resume the normal activity. Don't dwell on what upset you. Take your mind off the problem and go on. Keep in mind you'll have to practice this technique for a short time until it becomes automatic.

If you are under stress, you also can be affected by the foods you eat. According to a scientific study reported in *Epidemiological Journal, 1978, Volume 107,* people were monitored according to their personalities (Type A or B). They found the Type A nervous individuals had a higher death rate from heart disease than the calm, relaxed individual (Type B). As a result, it was assumed the higher death rate was due to the high stress levels involved.

When they decided to check on diet, the scientists were amazed to find the Type A individuals were eating 20% more cholesterol and 10% more saturated fats than the Type B individuals. They "theorized" that possibly it was the food that led to severe heart conditions.

Later, they conducted a follow up study in Framingham, Massachusetts, and to everyone's surprise they were unable to reproduce the same results. This time the Type B personalities had the higher death rate because now they were eating more fat and cholesterol than the Type A person. Stress can be very harmful for an individual with a heart condition. But, if you follow the

Healthy Aging Plan, you'll find when you get upset or stressful that you'll be more in control and feel more relaxed. Your circulation will be better and stress will not affect you so dangerously.

I'd like to share with you a typical case of a person with stress related problems: A gentleman age 53 and married. His chief complaint was fatigue. When he'd wake up in the morning he could hardly get himself out of bed. He was always tired and lacked energy. He also had difficulty concentrating and had a decrease in sexual energy.

In talking with him, we learned he was a CPA, a very stressful job according to him. We've found, though, most professions - doctor, real estate agents, and housewives - are all under stress! He had been at the same job for 20 years. He worked 10 to 12 hours per day; five to six days a week and he often brought work home with him. We would call this man a "workaholic." Here, though, work itself didn't seem to be the cause of stress. We checked further to find what could be causing his complaints. When this patient would become upset or find himself under a great deal of stress, he would use medications such as valium to calm his nerves. Valium is now considered one of the most commonly used prescription drugs in this country, with sales over $400,000,000. He also used Diazide and Dalmane for his blood pressure.

He also smoked about 40 cigarettes per day, drank a large glass of wine daily and five whiskey cocktails per week. He also drank eight to ten cups of coffee per day. He exercised only sporadically, and slept only about five to six hours per night. Considering the large amounts of coffee he consumed (about 1,250 milligrams of caffeine), it was surprising he could sleep at all!

He was overweight about 35 pounds and had a "typical" understanding of nutrition. His usual breakfast consisted of toast with butter, coffee, eggs and sausage. For lunch he would eat steak, french fries and pie. Dinner would be more meat, vegetables and dessert. Later, he'd snack on nuts, cheese, potato chips and alcoholic drinks. He used salt on his food, and about 16 teaspoons of sugar with whole milk in his coffee every day. He ate all the wrong foods daily, and rarely ate fruits, vegetables or cereals.

We also learned he ate about six eggs per week. Remember that since the body can only get rid of 100 milligrams of cholesterol per day, he had a severe build-up. His cholesterol level was 420! That is very, very high, as you know. It should be 100 plus your age, and never over 160. His triglycerides were 260 because of the fatty foods he was eating.

When questioned about his sexual problems, he said he was "just too tired, because I'm 53 years old. What do you expect?" Many people believe that as we get older, we're supposed to slow down. Our patient thought it was inevitable that with old age we become decrepit and incapable of living life to the fullest.

We shared our approach with him and showed him how to reduce the stress in his life. The great news is he reduced his cholesterol and triglyceride levels, lost weight and increased his energy level. Within a short time, his sex life was back to normal, also. As you can see, there are many benefits to eating properly, exercising and reducing stress!

**Supplements to help regulate blood pressure:** Bilberry, Black Cohosh, Cascara Sagrada, Cayenne, CoQ10, Ho-Shou-Wu, Siberian Ginseng, Una de Gato, Hawthorn berry, Garlic, Parsley, Cayenne, Valerian, Potassium citrate, Magnesium glycerophosphate, Golden Seal, Ginger, Siberian Ginseng, and Melatonin, liquid ionic minerals.

**Supplements to reduce stress and cortisol:** DHEA, alfalfa, Bee Pollen, Black Cohosh, Blue Vervain, Cayenne, Garlic, Parsley, Gotu Kola, Hawthorn Berry, Norwegian Kelp, Passion Flower, Pau d' Arc, St John's Wort, Stevia, Suma, B complex, grape seed extract, Una de Gato.

# XVII

∞

# CANCER: Stomach, Liver, & Leukemia

---

Cancer is probably one of the most feared diseases that affects our population. It claims over 400,000 lives each year and one out of four adults will contract cancer and die from this serious disease. It is the second leading cause of death in this country, after atherosclerosis or hardening of the arteries.

We have reviewed information about the causes of cancer and we now know a great deal about how to prevent it. Within the last few years both the *National Cancer Institute* and the *American Cancer Society* have published some of the largest documented reports (nearly 600 pages) following the many studies conducted by medical research departments across the country. These reports tell us over 54 percent of cancers are preventable through nutritional dietary changes. Unfortunately, there is very little financing to educate the public about nutrition, and most people have not heard about these anti-cancer reports. There is no way for a pharmaceutical company to patent the diet or for any other private groups to gain the finances to pay for newspaper, TV and radio publicity and education for the prevention of cancer. Unless the government sponsors massive education campaigns, it is up to us then, to spread the word and let people know there are several ways to avoid many types of cancer.

First we must understand what cancer is. Cancer is considered a mutation of the cells as they develop and grow. The actual function of the cell is altered in its capability to function as a normal cell. For example, under normal circumstances a liver cell reproduces another liver cell. But, during the production of additional cells, if the cell mutates and loses its ability to function as a viable liver cell, and eventually reproduces repeatedly, a tumor will form. A tumor is a growth or a group of cells that have no proper function in the body. They absorb energy and eat the body alive by replacing the function of essential organs.

While cancer mutations do occur from environmental factors, we are now learning a far greater cause of mutations is the basic oxygen-carrying capacity of the body. Dr. Otto Warburg of Germany, two time Nobel Prize winner, found a relationship between low oxygen levels and cancer. His work was later carried on by Dr. Goldblat, who conducted a series of fascinating experiments dating back to the 1950's. He took cardiac cells from an actual heart, had them reproduced and these heart cells were then put into two separate test tubes. One group of cells was deprived of oxygen while the other group was provided proper oxygen and hemoglobin to maintain its life.

In the group of cells **deprived of oxygen**, most of the cells died as you would expect. Yet, some cells survived and those surviving cells mutated, or changed their chromosomal makeup. These mutated cells became malignant. During one year's time, they injected these cells into animals and all the animals **died of cancer**! When doctors compared the malignant cells to the same original cardiac cell that **received proper oxygen** and hemoglobin after a period of two years, they found there were no malignant cells present in the test tube. They injected the cells into animals and **no** cancers developed. We have found, therefore, oxygen deprivation is a principal cause of mutated cells.

What could cause oxygen deprivation in the human body? We know high fat levels in the diet deprive the body of oxygen, while the low-fat Healthy Aging Plan will increase the amount of oxygen. Another way to fight cancer would be to increase your oxygen levels using exercise. One group of 1,000 long distance runners was found to have only 1/7 the cancer deaths of the general population. We have also discovered through autopsy report when blood vessels are examined, blockages of plaque or clots of cholesterol are present. Downstream of the blockages, where there is not enough oxygen reaching the cells, mutations occur or cancer develops. You need to reduce your cholesterol consumption to reduce the chance of plaques and cancer.

There are several different causes of cancer. If we look throughout the world, we discover **stomach cancer**, for example, is very high in Japan. But, when the Japanese migrate to the United States, the first generation has a one-third lower stomach cancer rate. Over time they become "Americanized" and adopt the American lifestyle, and eventually the stomach cancer rate is almost non-existent.

What is it about the Japanese diet or lifestyle that causes stomach cancer? We can identify several factors. First, the Japanese pickle their fish to preserve it in sodium nitrates, and we know these can turn into nitrosamines. Since there is a low vitamin C content in the Japanese diet, and nothing to prevent these nitrosamines from forming, we then have potential stomach cancer.

The second, and probably the greatest cause of stomach cancer in the Japanese, is the fact they used white rice coated with talcum powder. Talcum powder is mined in the same place as asbestos. If you can imagine, they used this talcum powder on the rice for cosmetic purposes - it made the rice look whiter. The result is they have had a tremendously higher rate of stomach cancer. Fortunately, the Japanese banned the use of talcum powder in rice by the end of the 1980's. Other forms of rice, brown and Chinese white rice, for example have no talcum powder.

The third factor for the Japanese is their excessive use of salt. They use 20 to 30 grams of salt per day, which may aggravate the stomach lining.

If we examine the Japanese rate of **colon cancer**, we discover they have a much lower rate of colon cancer per every hundred people. However, those Japanese who migrated from Japan to the United States, develop colon cancer at a rate of two and one-half times greater than their relatives of the same genetic race. If we compare the rate in Japan to the United States population as a whole, we find over four to five times the rate of colon cancer in the U.S. If the Japanese people adopt all the typical U.S. habits and food patterns, they develop colon cancer. Colon cancer, we have discovered is related to dietary factors. It's related to a lack of fiber and an overconsumption of fat in the diet, and we'll discuss that in more detail a little further on.

**Pancreatic cancer** is also somewhat low in Japan and much higher in the U.S. There is some correlation now with high fat diets and pancreatic cancer.

**Leukemia** is a cancer in which an overproduction of a certain type of white blood cell crowds out the function of other cells. There is an increase in leukemia in this country. Leukemia is also much higher in the U.S. than other countries. In the journal "*Science*" (Vol. 213, 1981), it was reported more than one third of the all U.S. dairy cows were infected with leukemia viruses. When virus infested milk were fed to chimpanzees, the experimental animals developed leukemia and die. Perhaps the fact the U.S. consumes more dairy products than all other nations combined accounts for this higher rate of leukemia in the U.S. There is also some early indication excessive fat levels may lead to many cases of leukemia. While leukemia can be treated with certain types of therapies, once a person develops cancer of any sort, it becomes a very serious situation.

Some doctors believe the body becomes acidic from consuming meat, milk, sugar and wheat grains. To restore alkaline blood you must eat more vegetables, basmati rice, barley greens, sprouts, sprouted bread, beans, hummus, lentils, soaked nuts, tomatoes, avocados and sour apples. Natural path Doctor, Robert Young believes that this approach will prevent the overgrowth of microorganisms, parasites, and cancer including leukemia.

Nathan Pritikin died at the age of 69 by taking his own life after a treatment for interferon failed and depressed his liver and kidney function. The leukemia was kept under control by his diet and exercise for a full 27 years. He did drink nonfat milk. Could this have caused the leukemia? Another theory is that an exposure to radiation treatment for a skin condition may have contributed to his leukemia. Pritikin had reluctantly agreed to undergo these x-ray treatments. He was exposed to 88 radiation doses (rads) on January 12, 1957 and three days later received the same dosage, with an additional 44 rads on February 16.

Two days later, a blood test showed he had an elevated white count and one year later he was told he had monoclonal macroglobulinemia. This is a condition that elevates the levels of globulins, or aggregated proteins and white blood cells that form clumps in the bloodstream. This is a blood disorder that in later stages can become leukemia. Nathan Pritikin was one of the great researchers and pioneers in the wellness industry. His program worked for so many tapes of diseases. He did reverse his own heart disease, and outlived the predictions by 24 years of only 3 years of life left, after the type of leukemia he was diagnosed with. We will never know if any further changes in his diet would have helped. He wanted to make sure the American public accepted the diet. From birth, dairy products are culturally ingrained in all of us.

There are several different mutations that can occur from various types of carcinogens. Recently we have discovered smoking food or charbroiling meat, especially higher fat cuts of meat, will increase the rate of carcinogenic property. For example, one pound of smoked mutton or lamb contains the equivalent of 250 cigarettes in carcinogenic properties. A quarter pound of charbroiled hamburger would contain more than a 50 cigarette equivalent. It's very upsetting for me to see certain hamburger chains promote fund raising activities to discover the cause of cancer, and yet children rush to these hamburger stands and potentially increase their risk of cancer dramatically.

The mutations that occur from benzo pyrene are a result of the fat dripping down onto the hot surface underneath and pyrolyzing, or changing chemically, and seeping back into the meat, where it remains. When you eat the meat, you ingest these carcinogenic properties. My suggestion is you prepare your meat differently. For example, when you select lower fat meats, such as chicken, fish or turkey, it's best to cook them in a casserole so the meat isn't in direct contact with a hot surface. If you use other types of cooking processes, such as a microwave, there is an avoidance of this benzo pyrene buildup.

Another cause of cancer that we have identified is related to an aflatoxin, which is a powerful carcinogen that is excreted from a fungus called Aspergillus flavus. This fungus generally grows on peanuts and other types of foods on occasion. Peanuts, though, are the most significant source. In Mozambique, where most of their diet is composed of peanuts, they have one of the highest rates of liver cancer in the world. You might think it's very unfortunate this poor group of people has such a high rate of liver cancer. Yet, when "Consumer Reports" analyzed over 14 different brands of peanuts and peanut butter, they found conclusively every brand of peanut butter had aflatoxin in it. Just because you eat peanut butter doesn't mean you'll develop liver cancer, since it is dose related. But, after several years of use, you very well could.

One study was done on starving Indian children who had been shipped peanut flour. They unknowingly ate the peanut flour that was contaminated with aflatoxin. It was found just three parts per million of aflatoxin over a 30-day period led to cirrhotic liver and death.

**Liver cancer** is on the increase in the United States today, and I'm always concerned when children are sent to school with their peanut butter and jelly sandwiches. We suggest you switch to almond butter or cashew butter, or any other kind of nut or seed. Peanuts are not a nut or seed at all, but a legume. They grow underground. All other nuts and seeds grow on top of land on vines or trees, and are rarely found to have fungus.

However, because peanuts do grow underground, they have a moist shell. It absorbs the moisture from the soil, and when it is pulled up from the ground, it's a fertile bed for this fungus, Aspergilus flavus, to grow. Even if you cook the peanuts, roast them, etc., it does not get rid of the aflatoxin. You may kill the fungus, but the aflatoxin is the excretion product, and it remains. Again, we highly recommend you reduce the use of peanuts. Occasionally would be fine, but don't use them regularly. All other nuts and seeds are safer to use, but because of their high fat content, only use them in small quantities (up to two ounces per day).

To cleanse your body and restore your immune system to prevent or fight cancer consume at least two or three raw vegetable, sprout, fruit drinks a day. Take supplements, herbs, phytochemicals, enzymes and restore your biochemical hormone levels. Avoid excess fat and cholesterol or protein. And take daily walks.

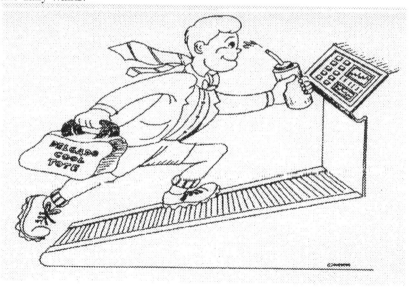

# XVIII

∞

# Breast Cancer Prevention

---

The principal cause of many cancers is fat in the diet. In studies comparing the amount of fat eaten in different countries, those who eat the most fat - Germany, United States and Denmark - have the highest rate of breast cancer as compared to countries like Thailand, Japan and Spain. Fat intake is closely linked to cancer development, according to Dr. Ernest Wynder, who is the world expert on breast cancer development. Dr. Wynder reported in the December, 1969 issue of *"The Cancer Report,"* "One can plot the incidence of breast cancer against any number of environmental factors. The one correlation that shows up well and may be of etiological significance is between breast cancer and the fat intake of women in various countries of the world."

Excessive dietary fat is the principal cause of breast cancer, which is the number one cause of death in women, age 35 to 55. It takes even more lives than hardening of the arteries or heart disease. This is unfortunate because often breast cancer can be prevented. For example, in Japan those people following a low fat diet have a very low incidence of breast cancer. Those few who do develop breast cancer are usually found in the inner city where they eat a higher fat diet. When Japanese who follow a low fat diet migrate to Hawaii, studies show they develop six times the rate of breast cancer as they increase the fat on the Hawaiian diet. We know breast cancer is not hereditary. If it were, the Japanese would have the same rate of cancer in all their genetic race, no matter where they lived.

There are three types of non-ʻcancerous lumps commonly found in womens breasts. Fibrocystic disease is defined as "lumpy breasts without cancer" and affects half of all women. Fibrodenomas are round, solid, "marble-like" and freely movable, appearing in the late teens and early twenties. They do not disappear by themselves and may enlarge during pregnancy and lactation. These fibro-adenomas are usually benign. A few studies show avoidance of caffeine for at least six months may remove the discomfort and shrink the fibrocystic lumps.

The second kind of non-cancerous lump appears between the ages of 30 to 39. They may fluctuate in size with the menstrual cycle; often they are sore or tender, appearing as an unusually distinct area, and are due to normal variations of breast tissue.

The third type of benign lumps are called cysts, which are firm, fluid-filled sacs and are usually painful. These appear around age 40. 90% of women develop cysts if they have used oral contraceptives longer than two to four years.

## CANCEROUS LUMPS

Cancers are hard lumps, usually, not tender and may be either movable or fixed to the skin or underlying tissue. In post-menopausal women, past the age of 45, a newly detected lump such as this should be biopsied. A mammogram is not sufficient to tell if the lump is malignant and cancerous (composed of mutated cells which spread and grow).

The forerunner to cancer is a condition of "hyperplasia" that means "overgrowth." In this situation, cells lining the milk ducts change their appearance, multiply and build up in a cluster inside the duct. In this early stage, a lump is not yet present and the build up of cells does not inevitably lead to cancer. This whole process is reversible up to this point. But, as the condition progresses, the cells may increase in size while becoming more irregular in appearance. Eventually, abnormal cells may plug the duct and then go on to break out of the duct, turning into an invasive cancer.

From autopsy findings, we can predict that of the 30% of women who develop hyperplasia, most them will not get cancer. Yet many women undergo mastectomies (total removal of breast tissue) as if the condition was cancer. This is a tragedy leading to unnecessary psychological suffering and physical disfigurement. This needless surgical approach also distorts the treatment statistics by including women who really didn't have cancer to begin with and mixing them in with true cancer cases. This results in false claims by surgeons of improved life expectancy. Incredibly, some women undergo preventive mastectomies simply because a relative had a history of breast cancer. Not long ago, I came across an article in the LA Times that was very upsetting. It reported some women were trying surgery as a preventive measure against breast cancer. I read the subheading and it stated, "Sharon Hughes - I haven't regretted it at all." She was encouraged to have a mastectomy - removal of the breast tissue - because her relatives had breast cancer, and although she showed no signs of the cancer at all, she volunteered to have this surgery done! If the physician in charge had been aware breast cancer is not hereditary, but is related to a high fat diet, she would have had a much better life knowing she could have prevented cancer naturally. We have seen no change in the survival rate in 1988, compared to the survival rate as far back as 1950. Surgery, radiation and chemotherapy have almost failed to make any difference.

Early detection with mammogram doesn't solve the problem either, because a breast tumor must be about the size of a pea before it shows on a mammogram. By that time, the tumor has been growing for at least ten years (*Guilliano, P., Cancer; 39:2697, 1977*). In 90% of the cases, the cancer cells have already entered the bloodstream and started to spread to the other organs of the body. So, early detection, followed by mastectomy, chemotherapy and radiation usually will not cure the woman because cancer of the breast doesn't kill. However, the spread of cancer to the brain, liver or lungs would most likely take the life 10 to 20 years later.

Women on a high fat diet menstruate as early as age 12 and begin menopause by age 50. By comparison, women in Thailand and Japan on a traditional low-fat, high starch complex carbohydrate diet start menstruation after age 26, begin menopause at age 46 and have the lowest rate of breast cancer in the world. This was true particularly before 1945. Since WWII, the Japanese diet has become higher in fat. When women from Thailand and Japan migrate to the U.S. and eat a high fat diet, they lose their immunity to breast cancer, developing equally high levels as American women. We know breast cancer is not genetic. It is related to fat in the diet.

Women on a low-fat diet have lower ideal estrogen levels, have lighter and shorter menstrual periods and have less or no pain associated with premenstrual syndrome. Lower estrogen levels reduce the formation of fibroid tumors in the muscular tissue of the uterus. Women with breast cancer have been given Tomoxifen hormone (antiestrogen drug), which has been shown to shrink tumors and improve survival as the estrogen levels are reduced. We also see a lessening of the pain and lumps of fibrocystic breast disease. Contrary to popular belief, we know breast cancer is not caused by a blunt object striking the breast.

We have also discovered malignant cells are unable to manufacture their own cholesterol (normal cells produce as much cholesterol as needed). Yet, when we analyze malignant tumor cells, they have even more cholesterol and fat than normal cells. The cancer cell needs to get its cholesterol from the host, and if you eat foods containing cholesterol, you will provide a generous supply. When we remove cholesterol from the diet to less than 50 mg. a day on the Healthy Aging Plan, the cancer tumors may shrink in size and disappear. A cancer cell can take the cholesterol and metabolize it into estrogen. It then uses the estrogen to stimulate growth in the surrounding tissue to spread throughout the body. Women or men can develop breast cancer if given female synthetic estrogens, because estrogen stimulates the sex organs and produces abnormal growth.

Cancer experts Dr. Ernest Wynder and Dennis Burkitt, M.D. believe a reduction of fat, cholesterol and protein, and an increase in fiber and phytochemicals in the diet may prevent breast cancer. They believe excess fat from oils, cheeses, meats and milk in the diet increases the production of bile acids in the intestines. This releases **excess estrogen** and **prolactin** hormones that may promote the development of breast cancer. Excess fatty acids in the breast tissue increase the production and secretion of the hormone prolactin, which can increase naturally during pregnancy. However, prolactin in excessively high levels has been correlated with the high rate of breast cancer. Women who have breast cancer generally have high prolactin hormone levels.

**Chasteberrry herb** reduces prolactin release and may suppress tumor growth. This herb may help because prolactin regulates growth of breast cells and the amount of circulating estrogen. High fat foods reach the intestines where bacteria produce even more estrogen. High levels of estrogen increases the growth of breast tissue and the risk of tumors. Breast cancers produce unusually large amounts of prostaglandins (10 times more than normal breast tissue does). This hormone-like substance also is increased in the body when we consume large amounts of processed essential fatty acids found in polyunsaturated vegetable oils such as corn, sunflower or safflower oil.

We have discovered, fortunately, women with high prolactin and estrogen hormone levels who reduce fat in their diet can reduce their prolactin and estrogen to safer levels within thirty days. This reduces the risk of breast cancer by 90%, according to Dr. Ernest Wynder. If you are trying to avoid this dread disease, breast cancer, switch to our low-fat, water rich complex carbohydrate diet.

We believe the risk of breast cancer can be reduced by as much as 90% in only 30 days time following a Healthy Aging Plan approach - less than 20% calories from fat and more than 70% calories from complex carbohydrates.

The regular daily exercise plan we recommend also may reduce the risk of breast cancer by increasing oxygen levels and reducing the circulating triglyceride fats in the blood.

A high fiber diet also may increase the excretion of estrogen by 2 to 3 times in the feces as compared with low fiber diets of animal products. Women who eat meat have 50% more estrogen in their bloodstream than vegetarian women. Obesity increased the production of estrogen and the risk of breast cancer. The Healthy Aging Plan can help you to reach your ideal body weight.

A small, but growing number of women are switching to our low-fat diet approach for treatment to control and possibly reverse cancerous tumors. It is unfortunate research money has only been given to large drug companies for chemotherapy (which has been unsuccessful in women who get breast cancer after menopause), to surgeons comparing which surgery is best and to mammography detection centers.

We strongly advise all women diagnosed with breast cancer to follow a low-fat diet. One out of every ten American women will get breast cancer (120,000 new cases annually and increasing). Major cancer societies now recommend following our type of plan. There have been cases documented of women overcoming cancer, and diet has been the key factor. If your physician is unfamiliar with our type of approach, California now has an informed consent law that requires a physician to explain alternative methods to surgery and we could offer advice on these different methods.

Alternative treatments for **breast cancer** usually include:

1. **Blended drinks** consuming at least two servings (48 oz each) a day of - sprouts, veggies, and fruit. Large **salads** (with nonfat dressings) at least once or twice a day. Consume at least 80% of your diet from raw food, 20% cooked food- Brown rice or basmati rice and other complex carbohydrates. Avoid all fat, oil, cholesterol foods meats, dairy, eggs.

**2. SUPPLEMENTS:**

**Hormone balance**: (if tested deficient on saliva, urine & blood) added progesterone cream daily, melatonin (sublingual), DHEA(spray or liposome cream), homeopathic human growth factor IGF-1, soy protein isolate, Suma (Brazilian Ginseng), Damiana, straw oats (Avena Sativa) and Saw Palmetto.

**Digestive Enzymes**-in capsules (Amylase, Protease, Lipase, Cellulase) consumed with cooked food.

**Herbs**- Aged Garlic Extract (allium sativa), Ginkgo Biloba, Una de Gato, Barley greens, chlorophyll, Bayberry, catnip, chickweed, fenugreek, getian, golden seal, irish moss, myrrh, blue vervain, comfrey, St. John's Wort, yellow dock, cyani, mandrake, fennel, Milk thistle, grapefruit, pectin, acerola, echinacea, burdock, dandelion, cayenne, chaste berry.

**Phytochemicals**- PhytoGen ( soy phytochemicals rich in genistein), Phyto Veggie & fruit capsules, Indoles (cruciferous vegetables) Bioflavonoids, Fructooligosaccharide (cellulose, legume apple pectin).

**Antioxidants**-Grape seed (OPC), Peruvian cat's claw-Uncaria Tomentosa

**Minerals**-ionic elements, calcium, magnesium, zinc, selenium, potassium

**Vitamins**- Multi-vitamin formulas derived from whole food complexes A, E, C, B-complex, B-12

**Essential fatty acids**- Evening primrose & flax seed

**Shark cartilage extract-Glucosamine**

**Fiber**- Cholesterade (Gum Arabic), Oat bran, Metamucil (psyllium).

3.**Far-Infrared-Wave** therapy (socks, sports wraps, seat pads, comforter).

4. **Exercise** & daily walks 30 minutes or more per session

5.Be resourceful, **positive state of mind**- ask power questions, enjoy comedy, funny movies, supportive friends, pray and attend to your spiritual life.

# XIX

# Colon, Lung, & Prostate Cancer

The foods we eat in the United States can cause cancer. **Colon cancer**, for example, is common in the average American. When you eat a high fat diet, there is so much bile acid produced that a bacteria called anaerobic bacteria grows and lives off this bile acid in an oxygen-less environment. Nearly one-third of your total bowel movement is made up of this anaerobic bacteria if you eat the typical American diet. These bacteria give off an excretion called deoxycolic acid, which is a proven carcinogen. This is one of the main reasons the American population is experiencing this increase in the rate of colon cancer.

Many people undergo colostomies to remove the colon, and this is very unfortunate because this type of disease is preventable. When you switch to a low-fat diet, the anaerobic bacteria can no longer live off the excess bile acid. These harmful anaerobic bacteria are pushed out of the body and replaced by good bacteria, called aerobic bacteria, which live in the presence of oxygen. In addition, the high fiber foods are soothing the digestive tract, which increases the intestinal content and actually push out any carcinogenic properties from the body. Remember, if your body passes stools every day, instead of every three days to two weeks, the potential for cancer development is reduced. In countries where they eat the most meat, like New Zealand, United States, Canada and the United Kingdom, they have the highest rate of colon cancer, nearly 40 times higher than in countries like Columbia, Hungary, Nigeria and Japan.

What is being done to prevent and minimize the recurrence of colon cancer in hospitals? An unfortunate example showed us the desperate need for change when former President Ronald Reagan had surgery for colon cancer.

He was served a hamburger just before his pre-surgery fast, and his first three meals after removal of the cancerous polyp from his colon were: eggs, bacon and buttered toast for breakfast, chicken broth and a cheeseburger for lunch and salmon for dinner - all in the hospital!

In the early 1950's in Japan, we discovered the rate for colon cancer was very low, less than 3 deaths per 100,000. Yet after World War II, with the dramatic change in their lifestyle, and accompanied by the increase of meat, eggs, fat and milk, there was a significant increase of three to four times the rate of colon cancer. This shows again how colon cancer is related to our lifestyle and the foods we eat.

Of the different types of cancer, **lung cancer** is the number one cause of death - nearly 70,000 people die every year. Cigarette smoking makes the lungs look black, charred and increases the mutagenic properties.

However, **cholesterol** is a key factor in the development of lung cancer according to an amazing piece of research by Dr. Jeremiah Stamler. He compared thousands of cigarette smokers, categorized them as moderate or heavy smokers and found those people with the highest cholesterol levels developed lung cancer. This was a shocking discovery.

What did cholesterol have to do with lung cancer? It was always assumed cigarette smoking was the principal cause. In fact, Dr. Stamler showed if a person had a cholesterol level under 150, it made no difference whether the person was a smoker or not. Usually, they did not develop lung cancer. Yet, if their cholesterol was 225-250, or higher, the rate went up to two thousand deaths - a nearly 2000% increase over cholesterol level under 150. If the cholesterol level was over 275, the rate skyrocketed to almost 4,000 deaths. The higher the cholesterol level, the higher the rate of lung cancer.

The correlation between cholesterol and lung cancer has finally been discovered. The lymphocytes (little white blood cells) back up against cancer cells and inject a substance that causes these cancer cells to burst and destroy themselves, while the macrophages (bigger white blood cells) engulf and digest cancer cells. In other words, white blood cells actually can eat viruses and cancer cells. It's been found the body may have developed cancer several times during your lifetime. However, if your white blood cells are active enough, they will protect you and save your life. If you have a high cholesterol level, though, we've discovered the white blood cells become paralyzed (inactive). If a cancer is triggered, for example, by cigarette smoking, asbestos, low oxygen levels in the body or some external factor, the cancer will start to grow. Because the white blood cells are paralyzed, the cancer grows and proliferates until it forms a large tumor and takes your life.

Excess cholesterol causes another problem. Cancerous tumors convert cholesterol into estrogen. As we stated earlier, increased amounts of estrogen in a man or woman's body stimulates the rapid growth of cancer into the surrounding tissue. Cancer cells cannot produce their own cholesterol as normal cells do, they must rely on the host. Studies have shown if you deprive cancer cells of cholesterol, you can shrink the tumor. According the *American Journal of Clinical Nutrition (Vol. 37, 1983)*, the risk of developing lung cancer was directly related to the amount of cholesterol consumed in all five major ethnic groups found in Hawaii. Those people who consumed the least amount of cholesterol rarely developed lung cancer, while those people who consumed the most cholesterol from eggs, meat, organ meats and dairy products had the highest rate of lung cancer.

We know meat is very high in fat content. Also, there is a potential carcinogenic property in beef. Cattle grown on the feed lots grow more rapidly because of the 120 different chemicals given to them. What are these synthetic growth hormones, antibiotics and chemicals doing to your body? Isn't it likely some of them are turning into cancer? There are over 20 different chemicals used in our livestock today that have already been identified as carcinogenic. The FDA has banned one of them -DES. Although you may have heard DES causes **uterine cancer** nearly 20 years after use, they are still discovering quantities of DES in meat eaten by the public. It's suspected the cattle producers are still slipping DES, this growth hormone, into these animals illegally.

Cholesterol crystals are associated with **prostate cancer**. Over half the men past the age of 50 in the U.S. have enlarged prostate glands, resulting in obstruction of the urethra and the slowing of the urine. A simple infection of the prostate or a high fat diet can increase sex hormones leading to enlargement. A change of diet and antibiotics, if needed, will reduce the swelling to normal. But, if the enlarged prostate is found to have cholesterol crystals within, then this could develop into prostate cancer. A study of 106 cysts (cysts are cocoon encasings of fibroblasts spun by your body around foreign objects that your white blood cells were unable to remove) showed that only 5 were malignant with cancer. The five that were malignant were the only ones with cholesterol crystals.

Experiments have shown when animals were injected with a large amount of cholesterol dissolved in olive oil, it crystallized within the animal and caused malignant cysts to form. When olive oil by itself was injected, some cysts were formed, but no malignancies developed. Plastic cysts were then inserted under animals skin and within two weeks cocoons formed around the foreign object and malignant cells were found inside. If a plastic disc had scratches and holes drilled into it, and then was inserted into an animal, the cocoon formed, but no malignancies could be found. It was discovered the scratches and holes allowed capillaries to take hold and grow inside the cocoon and supply sufficient oxygen to the cells inside, thus preventing cancer. But, the smooth plastic disc and the cholesterol crystals (which are smooth) did not allow enough room for the capillaries to squeeze in as the fibroblasts spun their tight web. This deprivation of oxygen and food causes some cells to die and some to mutate to cancer.

In Canada, three individuals, average age 65 and older, were proven to have **prostate cancer**. This was verified by needle biopsy. In this procedure, they stick a needle into the prostate and remove cells for testing. The test samples were loaded with cancer. Instead of surgery, these three men volunteered to follow a program that advocated a low cholesterol diet and certain types of cholesterol lowering drug therapy. In essence, they lowered the cholesterol level, and within a period of one month to three years, the cancer had disappeared, confirmed by another needle biopsy. The prostate had shrunk to normal and there was no longer any sign of prostate cancer.

Cancer prevention can be accomplished through a series of steps. You need to reduce your dietary fat intake to under 20%. This is recommended by both the **National Cancer Institute** and the **American Cancer Society**. You need to cut cholesterol consumption to under 100 mg. per day. Remember, reduced cholesterol in the bloodstream can improve white blood cell activity, help reduce estrogen production to safe levels and lessen the chance of malignant cocoon formation. Reduce smoked, salt-cured or pickled foods. Switch to lean cuts of meat (chicken, fish or turkey) or, better yet, stop the use of all meats.

Stop cigarette smoking to reduce the exposure to carcinogenic chemicals and the loss of oxygen due to carbon monoxide. Next, reduce the use of alcohol. Excessive alcohol intake combined with smoking may be correlated to **esophagus cancer** (highest in France). Also, chewing tobacco is related to **cancers of the mouth**. Avoid pollutants, asbestos and additives as much as possible. Reduce the use of peanuts and peanut butter, switching to whole nuts (almonds, cashews, walnuts, etc.) and seeds (sesame, sunflower,etc.) instead.

Eat more fruits and vegetables containing beta-carotene. Beta-carotene foods (which convert into vitamin A as your body needs it) such as carrots, broccoli and brussels sprouts, have a preventive effect on cancer. Those people with high vitamin A levels have a lower rate of cancer than those with a low vitamin A level. Vitamin C rich foods like red bell peppers, chili peppers, broccoli and strawberries reduce the rate of nitrosamine formation and stomach cancers. Increase the use of whole grains for their fiber content to keep your intestinal tract clean and healthful.

The *National Cancer Institute* is correct in assuming most cases of cancer are preventable. We have seen the benefits of our type of program in the treatment of cancer. Please help us spread the word to your loved ones. Don't depend on current therapies alone; get a second opinion from one of our doctors.

Hospitals are currently using methods considered less effective for cancer therapy, which may have side effects and may depress your immune system and decrease survival time. For example, a major surgery such as mastectomy should be replaced by a less radical procedure -a lumpectomy, in most cases. This also would reduce the use of blood transfusions. Radiation treatment also may depress your immune system and increase the risk of metastatic disease, according to the medical journal *Lancet (2:1285, 1974)*. Chemotherapy, which is the use of drugs by injection or pills, has been ineffective in prolonging life after cancer develops (*Lancet, 2:307, 1984*). Lymph node irradiation and lymph node removal is now questioned because lymph nodes produce lymphocytes that help fight cancer, and removal or radiation of the lymph nodes is not beneficial. Finally, the high fat diet served in hospitals worsen the problem. We expect to change that. Don't you think you should start following the Healthy Aging Plan? If you have already started our program, stay with it and encourage your friends to start.

If you think prostate cancer is very easy to cure, you're wrong. It's one of the most serious types of cancers. Years ago, when I worked in physical therapy critical care, I remember a man who had prostate cancer. It was our job to exercise him and keep him as strong as possible. He would exercise up and down the halls and seemed perfectly healthy; the only way we knew he had prostate cancer was from medical tests. He was not provided any special nutritional low-fat diet. He ate the typical high fat hospital food. After only two weeks, he was so fatigued and weak he could barely get out of bed. Two days later he could barely raise his arm. The cancer had grown in the prostate so severely it took away all his energy and it killed him within three weeks.

Dr. Anthony Sattilaro, a physician and president of Philadelphia's Methodist Hospital, contracted a serious case of cancer. According to bone scans, Dr. Sattilaro was diagnosed in May, 1978 with cancerous tumors in his brain, shoulder, ribs and testicles. At first, they did a biopsy, then removed one of his ribs and found it was loaded with cancer. They started chemo-therapy (drugs) to kill the cancer, and his health decreased rapidly. They removed both his testicles and tried hormone therapy. Since Dr. Sattilaro was a physician in a large hospital, he had access to all the latest therapies and treatments for cancer, but the other doctors gave up and told him he probably would die shortly and he should get his life in order.

According to "Life Magazine" and a follow up book by Dr. Sattilaro, he left his post at the hospital, went for a drive and encountered two young men. He talked with them, told them he had cancer and was going to die. After listening to his story, these young men told the doctor about a special diet that seemed to help those with cancer to live. He didn't believe it at first, after all, he was a doctor and thought he knew everything about cancer therapy. Finally, Dr. Sattilaro decided to follow their suggestion and began following a program that encouraged eating whole grains, vegetables and beans, while avoiding all fats, dairy and animal products.

Because of his changing lifestyle, Dr. Sattilaro started to feel better and the pain throughout his body began to go away. Fourteen months later, a further bone scan revealed all the cancer had disappeared from his body. His body had cleaned itself. How? Dr. Sattilaro reports, with his colleagues, perhaps as his diet was purified, his white blood cells could finally gain enough strength to fight off this serious cancer. Years later I followed up with colleagues who knew of his amazing recovery. However, Dr. Sattilaro had passed on from cancer. His relatives said that he had gone off his diet and the cancer had reoccurred. The cancer never goes away completely. You must change you life style permanently for ongoing protection.

Henry Heimlich, MD, in an interview with Dr. John McDougall shared his belief that when cancer patients got severe febrile diseases like malaria that caused a **high fever**, which had otherwise found to be incurable, often disappeared. Over 700 cases were found to improve. This amazing way to *stimulate the immune system* may become a new treatment of the future. That is to induce malaria in cancer patients. Cancer is unable to produce it's own fever because the cancer cells are recognized as part of the body. We can trick the body to defend itself and later cure the malaria fever.

The ability to enhance the immune system by restoring a **slightly alkaline blood PH** can be done by avoiding acid producing meat, dairy, sugar and wheat grains, while consuming alkaline restoring sprouts, veggies, basmati rice, beans, and avocados. The diet should be over 80% raw food. Molds, yeast, fungus, bacteria, viruses, and cancer all decline when the body is maintained in a healthy state. **Use herbs** like echinacea, germanium, Red Clover, Una de Gato, Licorice, Pau d'Arco, Ginko, Aleo Vera, Cascara Sagrada, Native legend Tea, Cat's claw, Acidophilus (non-dairy), and Bee Pollen. **Hormones** of DHEA, and melatonin. **Antioxidants** of Grape seed (OPC), bioflavonoids, **Digestive Enzymes**, Phyto veggies & fruit capsules, ionic **minerals**, and Cholesterade **fiber**(Gum Arabic), psyllum, and oat bran.

A new technology developed by NASA for use on the space shuttle reentry tiles has found its way into wellness centers. In Japan**, Far Infrared Wave Technology** has been applied to use the body's own infrared waves to regulate the body temperature. A sleeping couple that uses a Far Infrared Wave (FIR) technology bed comforter where one likes it hot and the other cold, will find they both achieve the ideal sleeping temperature. FIR therapeutically applied (Seat pads, socks, sports wraps), can alter the pH in the human body by neutralizing the acid and restore proper alkaline balance to treat cancer, back pain, gout, asthma, diabetes, and rheumatism, per Japanese-studies.

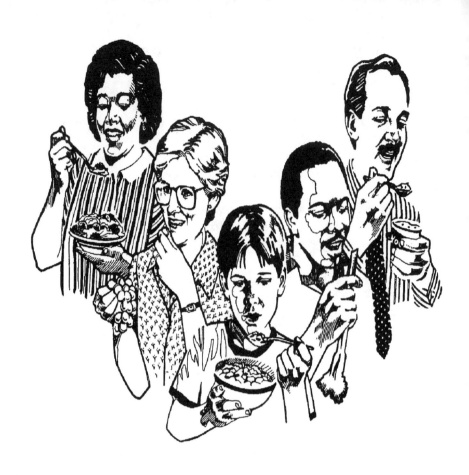

# XX

# Arthritis

---

Arthritis affects 25% of the United States population. That means 50,000,000 Americans suffer from this painful disease. It accounts for over a billion dollars lost every year through Social Security Disability payments issued to individuals unable to function because of this devastating disease. The Healthy Aging plan can stop the pain, and prevent further breakdown of the joints. Arthritis has many different causes.

One of the most painful forms is **gouty arthritis**, which generally affects the toe joint first, although it can affect nearly any joint in the body. Gout was very common in the Middle Ages and was at its highest rate in recorded history at that time. Their diet included large amounts of meat - at least six times per day; a typical dish was blackbird pie, a dish in which birds were actually baked in the pie shell!

A sample of blood viewed through a microscope from an individual with gout will reveal sharp crystals. These uric acid crystals attack the joints and cause destruction. It is interesting that these crystals do not destroy the joints directly. Your white blood cells play a role in this destruction.

If your uric acid level is over 7, it is very likely you will develop a gouty arthritis attack. Uric acid is a waste product of nucleic acid found in animal products and high protein foods. A diet high in protein, cheese, other dairy products and animal flesh will cause an elevation of uric acid. If the uric acid level in the bloodstream becomes too high, sharp crystals will form.

Your white blood cells know uric acid crystals should not be in the bloodstream. The white blood cells will begin to engulf these sharp crystals and try to dissolve them. Unfortunately, these crystals are one of the few things in nature the white blood cells cannot overpower. White blood cells can eat and dissolve cancer cells, various bacteria and foreign bodies in your intestinal lining, but they cannot digest uric acid crystals.

Within the white blood cells are little sacks called lysosomes that are the most powerful digestive juices in the human body. When the sharp uric acid crystals puncture the lysosomes, these juices dissolve the outer part of the white blood cell and release into the joint area and begin to dissolve the joint.

Gouty arthritis is one of the easiest problems to cure; you simply reduce the excess proteins in the diet and begin consuming more complex carbohydrates. Within 12 weeks, elevated uric acid levels will lower to a safe range because the crystals begin to dissolve as protein is reduced.

Blood pressure medications will create an artificial elevation of uric acid levels. When Zyloprim or Benamid are prescribed to lower these uric acid levels, other side effects result. It's better to correct the cause naturally and safely by diet.

**Rheumatoid arthritis** is a more serious form of arthritis. This also involves the white blood cells, but differently than described above. When there is a low oxygen level in the joint area, the white blood cells explode because of a lack of oxygen and release their strong digestive juices, which begin to dissolve the joints.

Medical studies have shown arthritics have a very low oxygen level in the joints. The reason for the low levels is a blockage of red blood cells in the blood vessels that occurs from consuming a high fat diet. A high fat diet is the principal cause of **rheumatoid arthritis**. The excess fat coats the red blood cells. These red blood cell "clumps" are now too large to squeeze through the capillaries, causing them to become blocked. Imagine how small red blood cells are - a head of a pin can hold five million! Normally, the red blood cells should bounce off each other; but, if there is a large amount of fat in the bloodstream, the red blood cells stick together and form clumps which then create blockages.

When a blockage occurs, the blood fluid keeps pumping and is forced into the surrounding tissues and causes edema. You can literally leave a finger mark or indentation in the skin area affected by edema. Many people with arthritis have edema, but are not aware of it because before edema is visible, one must have a build-up of over 60% fluid.

Edema is also caused by physical trauma. When one is hit on top of the head, a bump forms. This bump is comprised of fluid that accumulates to keep the tissues in place to reduce further destruction. This fluid is so low in oxygen the white blood cells begin to destroy themselves.

One example is "housemaid's knee." A person constantly on their knees will damage the joints. Edema will form because of the accumulation of fluids from trauma and a high fat diet. This fluid accumulation leads to arthritis of the knee because the white blood cells begin to destroy themselves. The same trauma can occur to a construction worker who continually uses a jackhammer to break concrete. The constant vibration leads to arthritis of the fingers.

But, it doesn't always have to be a trauma that leads to edema. We know women have a 200% higher incidence of arthritis than men. As fluids accumulate during the menstrual cycle, the edema concentration, combined with a high fat diet, will cause arthritis.

Another extremely painful type of arthritis is **osteoarthritis** and is the most difficult to treat. This form of arthritis occurs when the cartilage is damaged due to low oxygen levels. When the white blood cells begin to eat the cartilage, the cartilage seems to alter itself for protection and begins to form itself into bone matter. This will result in bone rubbing directly against bone.

Until recently the only help offered to the arthritis sufferer was anti-inflammatory drugs, including cortisone and aspirin. Although symptoms improve, the deterioration continues within the joints and additional side effects from the drugs may be experienced.

The side effect from aspirin is stomach damage. Cortisone has other side effects after long-term use, including muscle wasting, ulcers, fluid and fat gains. Some pain is reduced temporarily because these drugs suppress white blood cell activity, thus reducing the number of white blood cells left to release their digestive juices. Remember, though, your white blood cells also protect you from disease and infection. With this suppression, you are now susceptible to other problems.

Medical researchers at UCLA extracted white blood cells from the lymph system of patients to treat arthritis. Millions of white blood cells were drained until the symptoms of arthritis were reduced. The patients experienced temporary relief, until the white blood cell count returned to normal and the pain in the joints returned. As you can appreciate, just removing or immobilizing the white blood cells does not address the cause of the problem. We could control this disease if people would recognize arthritis is a result of the high fat foods we eat. For those who believe it is due to heredity, let's examine the Pima Indians.

These Indians live in Arizona, and as a group, consume one of the highest fat diets in our country. Because of this high fat diet, the Pima Indians recorded the highest rate of **arthritis** in our country, and they also have an extremely high rate of gallstones. **Gallstones** are a concentration of cholesterol in the gallbladder, along with an imbalance of polyunsaturated fats. Gallstones can be dissolved by reducing fat and cholesterol in the diet.

We say arthritis is not genetic because the blood relatives of the Pimas, the Tarahumara Indians, consume a high complex carbohydrate diet and have no incidence of arthritis or gallstones. If there were a genetic factor, these people would suffer the same problems.

There are many success stories about alleviating the symptoms of arthritis. One such story is about a ballet teacher, who was severely affected. Every morning she had to sit in a hot tub just to move. If she had no help to get to the tub, she would drag herself there. She started avoiding fats, she increased her complex carbohydrates to rid herself of the pain and stiffness. She was fortunate the arthritis had been caught and stopped before the joints had degenerated. There was some scar tissue and some knobby accumulation, but at least further damage was prevented. This woman returned to her teaching and conducted a ballet tour that was extremely important to her career. Later, she went back to school and became a nutritionist by the age of 53.

Another story is about the wife of a chiropractor, who was afflicted with a severe case of **rheumatoid arthritis** though she was only in her early thirties. Her pain and stiffness were eliminated following our recommendations regarding a Healthy Aging plan.

I met another woman before I became involved in nutritional research, however, who was not so fortunate. This woman had such a severe case of arthritis that just touching her body would cause tears to roll down her face. Her joints were so crippled her fingers and toes curled under. Her rheumatologist (doctor specializing in the treatment of arthritis) had prescribed several expensive drugs to no avail. Surgery was done on one knee joint and before success could be verified, surgery was performed on her other knee. Unfortunately, the left knee was left at a 45 degree angle. Her right knee also became totally immobilized after surgery. Her normal breakfast consisted of eggs with bacon and toast with butter. She ate one of the fattiest diets I've ever seen. It was never suggested to her she should change her diet, reduce the large amounts of butter, meat and cheese she was consuming.

The medical dictionaries that are currently available state there is no known cause for arthritis. It is believed by some people arthritis may be caused by some virus. Yet, if the people who prepared the medical dictionaries would do some research and read current literature, they would find the answers are already available. There are enough case studies and worldwide studies proving dietary changes can make arthritis a disease of the past.

To reduce the known arthritis forms, it is important to reduce fats in the diet. Begin by consuming more complex carbohydrates. Also, be sure to reduce salt in the diet, because salt causes additional fluid accumulation, which aggravates the arthritis. Exercise will help to reduce fat and fluid accumulation and stress reduction; relaxation techniques also will reduce arthritis symptoms.

If this doesn't give fully immediate relief within seven weeks, investigate allergies to foods. For example, avoid all dairy products, cheese, yogurt and nonfat milk included. In some people milk proteins are not completely digested. Large particles enter the bloodstream where allergic reactions can disrupt the white blood cells and the immune system. Even tiny amounts of milk added to cereal or coffee will cause massive destruction, pain and stiffness in some people.

One lady was cured of arthritis by avoiding all dairy products. However, after only one small serving of a milk product, the pain and stiffness struck her joints within 24 hours! It took her several days of dairy-free eating to recover.

Some people may be allergic to wheat, soybean, eggs, citrus fruit or potatoes. To determine your allergy, eat only brown rice, brown rice cereal or bread, non-citrus cooked fruits, yams and squash. Then gradually introduce one food at a time to test for one week. Eventually you'll discover what foods you must permanently avoid. This is called the "Elimination Diet Method." Then rotate the foods you know are safe, so you're not eating the same single foods all the time, to avoid becoming allergic to any of the safe foods.

A "rotation diet" is not as effective when you're still eating foods each week that you know you're allergic to. This does not work in long term treatment. Once you're allergic to certain foods, you'll continue to be allergic to those foods.

Have you heard the suggestion of taking oil to lubricate the joints? Be aware the fluid that lubricates joints is made up of carbohydrates - and oil contains no carbohydrates. The use of vegetable oil or cod liver oil will worsen arthritis!

The best approach to reducing **gouty, rheumatoid & osteoarthritis** is:
1) Improve circulation and reduce edema;
   a) Reduce fats, oils, cheese, fatty meat, etc. use only essential fatty acids from whole sprouted flaxseeds & Evening Primrose b) Reduce salt c) Aerobic exercise
2) Reduce protein (uric acid).
3) Physical therapy, including hot or cold therapy.
4) Restore female hormone balance using natural progesterone cream, DHEA, testosterone herbs Avena Sativa with exercise & a low-fat diet.
   (Osteoporosis may be the cause of pain that can worsen if the
   female hormones are out of balance.)
5) Eat complex carbohydrates, whole grain rice, beans, fruits & vegetables.
6) Lose weight if necessary.
7) Avoid dairy products for at least 6 months to note any
   improvement, and give your system time to clear allergies.
8) Identify allergy producing foods by the PRIME TEST/Fast-eliminate.
9) Use Herbs: Alfalfa, Black Cohosh, Burdock, Cayenne, Devil Claw, Echinacea, Ginkgo Biloba, Hawaiian Noni, Licorice, Pau d' Arco, Yucca, White Willow, Hydrangea, Sarsaparilla, parsley, Evening Primrose oil, long chain fatty acid cetyl ester, Calcium, magnesium, ionic minerals (92 organic mineral salts & trace).

# XXI

# Diabetes

---

There are ten million diabetics in the United States. They are at greater risk of heart attack, stroke, kidney damage, blindness and gangrene, with three times as high a death rate as do non-diabetics. A person is considered diabetic if the blood glucose level after fasting 8 to 12 hours exceeds 130 mg. on two separate occasions. Even after a very large meal, the blood sugar should not exceed 150 mg.

Symptoms of diabetes may include: fatigue, lack of energy, urination at night, and constant thirst (needing water every 15 to 30 minutes to dissolve the overflow of unused sugar in the blood and urine). Also, blurred vision (due to sugar accumulation in the lens of the eye) and weight loss (because of rapid burning of body fat due to your body's inability to use glucose).

Diabetes is mistakenly thought to be "well controlled" by insulin shots or pills. Diabetic drugs can control the blood sugar level, but the drugs have not helped to stop the rapid development of atherosclerosis associated with the diabetic condition. Diabetes is increasing in our country at the rate of 1.5 million new cases developing every year (a 15% yearly increase).

I vividly remember working in the physical therapy department of a hospital where I met a man named Charles. He was intelligent, kind and had a great sense of humor. Unfortunately, he could no longer continue his job as a university administrator, because he had become totally disabled by diabetes. He told me he had been at a party and had one drink, and nearly passed out. Everyone thought he was drunk, but later doctors confirmed he had developed diabetes. A year later, he suffered a stroke, and lost the ability to speak clearly (due to brain damage), lost control of his right arm, leg and bowels (he had to wear diapers). Charles became bedridden, and because of the constant pressure on the skin from lying in bed all day, he developed bedsores on his right leg and hip. The nurses tried to keep turning at regular intervals, because anyone who is weak and unable to roll over is in constant danger of bedsores.

Diabetes doesn't allow for proper healing of even minor sores, and before long the doctors had to amputate his left leg - his strong leg - opposite his stroke weakened leg. We were asked to give Charles whirlpool and ultraviolet light treatments for the bedsores on his hip and remaining ulcerated ankle, where you could now see bone and tendons. The doctors struggled to save his remaining leg, but it was no use.

I noticed every morning when I came to help Charles exercise that he was served 2 eggs, white toast with butter and bacon or sausage on the side. His lunches and dinners included large amounts of cheese, meat and dairy products. He was given only small amounts of vegetables and fruits, and even small amounts of whole grains or beans. I tried to tell my patients how important it was to reduce fat in the diet. However, patients in hospitals and convalescent homes are fed a diet based on outdated recommendations. I was unable to have the dietary departments change because I was told state laws had guidelines requiring the "four food groups." This could only be changed with doctors' orders and very few doctors in 1978 were prescribing a low-fat, high fiber diet for patients as treatment.

Now, several years later, we have shown the effectiveness of our program, and more doctors are recommending our approach to their patients. The fact remains, though, millions of people, and especially the ones you love and care about are still unaware of how to achieve this ideal health. Help us bring the Healthy Aging Plan to your community hospital. Contact the doctors and administrators and we can help them to meet the new 1999 federal guidelines for "Wellness Plans".

Two scientists, Burson and Yao, won the Nobel Prize after proving a person with diabetes produces as much insulin as a normal person (in 90% of the cases). From this information, we know diabetes is usually not caused by a lack of insulin. We have discovered the principal cause of diabetes is excess fat in the blood, which can desensitize the insulin, and the insulin is then unable to push glucose into the cells for energy. The fat accumulates in the blood from overeating fatty foods such as cheese, butter, margarine, oil, red meat and eggs, and from a lack of regular exercise.

You may develop a "**temporary case**" **of diabetes** if you have:

1) **FASTING** OVER 48 HOURS - You use your glucose in 12 hours, and then your body is forced to release fat in the blood for reserve energy, just as if you had eaten fat.

2) **FEVER** - Your body temporarily releases fat in the blood for up to 90 days when you have a fever.

3) **STRENUOUS EXERCISE** (beyond your capabilities) - This can use your body's storage of glucose, which would trigger the release of fat for replacement energy.

While this fat in the bloodstream can temporarily desensitize the insulin, you don't have to worry about occasionally testing diabetic in these short-lived, mild cases. Serious damage may only occur from years of poor diet or in people who can't produce insulin.

A severe form of the disease called "**insulin-dependent diabetes**" is caused by the inability of the pancreas to produce insulin in less than 10% of the people with diabetes. The pancreas can be damaged for the following reasons:

1) Excessive long-term use of **alcohol - Cirrhotic liver damage** from alcohol also can lead to the inability to handle fat, resulting in diabetes.
2) A **virus infection**, such as the mumps or the flu in some children.
3) **Overproduction of hormones** by adrenal, thyroid or pituitary glands.
4) An inherited **malfunction of the pancreas**.
5) Severe **allergic reaction** to dairy products, or from consuming other foods you may be allergic to. This can damage the pancreas.

In all of these cases, a low-fat diet with exercise can help you to avoid atherosclerosis, blindness and kidney damage that is usually associated with diabetes. You may reduce your need for insulin to body requirements (about 30 units per day), but you probably will need to take insulin for the rest of your life.

You probably will always need insulin if you were started on it before you were thirty years old. If you are very lean and take over 30 units of insulin per day, or if you are very lean and exercise a great deal (for example, run 15 miles/24 km per week or walk briskly 3 miles/5 km per day) and take over 20 units per day. On the other hand, if you are overweight and not very active, with your doctor's help through exercise and weight loss, you can gradually reduce your insulin dose. You may be able to stop your insulin injections with a suitable diet, such as the Healthy Aging Plan. UNDER NO CIRCUMSTANCES SHOULD YOU EVER ATTEMPT TO COME OFF INSULIN EXCEPT UNDER YOUR DOCTORS SUPERVISION.

In a 1935 study of 100 patients, Dr. Rabinowitz, placed half the patients on a low-fat diet (under 20%, as we recommend), and the other half on a high fat diet (56% fat). After the study, it was discovered those on a low-fat diet totally eliminated the need for injected insulin in 24% of the cases and reduced the need for insulin by over 58%. The group on the high fat diet was unable to reduce its insulin at all (less than 1%). The cholesterol levels were also dramatically reduced on the low-fat diet. Dr. Rabinowitz hypothesized it was the low cholesterol, low-fat diet that was the principal reason these diabetics did not develop heart disease, serious gangrene and other side effects, and he was right. He understood this idea back in 1935! Dr. Rabinowitz tried to convince the American public to change their diet, but no one would believe him. Everyone thought diabetes could not be controlled by diet and you would have to take insulin for the rest of your life.

Dr. James Anderson conducted another study investigating the cause of diabetes in 1979 at the University of Kentucky Medical Center. Dr. Anderson asked his patients to eat one pound of sugar every day for eleven weeks. Can you imagine eating a pound of sugar every day! That would be like eating one of those five-pound containers of sugar in less than a week's time! The rest of the diet was composed of only 5% fat. After the full eleven-week testing period, and after checking their blood sugar level weekly, not one person tested diabetic on the glucose tolerance test. The patients' sugar level always measured in the low range; it would have to be over 175 by glucose tolerance to test diabetic. The results were shocking because it was thought sugar caused diabetes.

Afterward, Dr. Anderson tried a diet high in fats (65% fat) with almost no fiber present. In less than two weeks time, every person tested diabetic. He then tried a diet of 45% fat without complex carbohydrates or fiber present and everyone tested diabetic again. He had discovered fat in the diet caused diabetes and not sugars. He then tested a diet with 40% complex carbohydrates and 43% fat. The blood sugar level was higher than the group eating the pound of sugar per day, but it did not get into the diabetic range because the complex carbohydrates with fiber have a protective factor on the insulin itself.

However, if you increase your fat intake for a long period, year after year, one day you'll probably test diabetic. It's assumed people past the age of 65 will eventually become diabetic. This doesn't have to happen. Studies show diabetes does not appear in cultures that follow a low-fat diet throughout their lives.

We strongly recommend you visit your doctor to have your blood sugar level checked. If after a fasting test, it's over 100, you're already testing diabetic. If it is 130 or higher, more than likely you're already diabetic. If after eating or having a glucose tolerance test, it goes over 180 and does not return below 100 mg., you are diabetic.

In a second study reported in The Medical Times, May 1980, Dr. Anderson altered the diet of 20 lean diabetics. He selected lean individuals because some doctors would tell their patients to lose weight and the diabetes would be gone. Dr. Anderson discovered weight loss alone wouldn't cure diabetes, although losing weight does help. The diabetics ate a 70% complex carbohydrate, high starch diet for two weeks. Dr. Anderson lowered the fat in the diet and had them eat Shredded Wheat, Grapenuts, crackers, whole wheat, rye bread, beans and raw fruit. The exciting results showed a reduction of insulin by 58% and cholesterol reduction by 30%. Diabetes Outlook also recommended the high complex carbohydrate, low-fat diet to avoid diabetes. The medical journals are coming out with more research showing a whole diet approach is better and safer to use than taking drugs or resorting to insulin.

Past treatments for diabetes have been varied and ineffective; in France they would give people a quarter pound of candy and small amounts of meat. Of course, it didn't help. In England, people were told to eat a high fat diet with no carbohydrates at all. Diabetics were told to eat fat, pork, blood and intestines, as rancid as they could bear. Unfortunately, this increased the death rate of the diabetics. Since they avoided carbohydrates, the doctors thought they were helping the problem!

There has been so much confusion in our country, too, about avoiding carbohydrates as treatment for diabetes. Yet, the Egyptians, 3,500 years ago, knew a low-fat, high complex carbohydrate diet was the best treatment for diabetics. It's written in their hieroglyphics: breads, berries and fruit. The Romans also knew this high fiber; low-fat diet would control diabetes. Dr. Kelly West, world-renowned endocrinologist, has reported over 62% of the adult-onset diabetics could be off insulin and back to normal on this low-fat, high complex carbohydrate diet. Dr. Kempner also reported similar results at Duke University.

The benefits of the complex carbohydrates include increased endurance, greater energy, lowering of blood fats, reduced cholesterol and triglycerides, increased fiber or bulk to the stools and control of the blood sugar level. We know exercise also reduces the blood glucose level by reducing fat in the blood and improves the sensitivity of insulin, whereas bed rest and inactivity causes high blood sugar levels. We also know hypo-glycemia, which formerly was treated by a high protein diet, is best controlled by the water rich, complex carbohydrates. The Healthy Aging Plan can give you enough blood sugar to control and maintain a high, even source of energy. Eat more potatoes, fresh fruits and vegetables and you'll be rid of hypoglycemia.

In summary, to avoid diabetes we recommend you eat more complex carbohydrates (grains, starches, beans, vegetables and fruit) and reduce the foods that cause diabetes - fats, oils, cheeses and meats. You also should increase aerobic exercise (30 minutes daily is sufficient), visit the doctor regularly if you are on insulin to change the dosages as needed and reduce sugar intake to avoid hypoglycemia (although sugar is not the cause of diabetes, it may lead to hypoglycemia). The major agencies - the Diabetic Association and the Cancer Institute now agree with the Healthy Aging Plan to reduce fat to under 20%, increase complex carbohydrates to over 70% and reduce cholesterol intake.

**Supplements** to reduce diabetes include Aged Garlic Extract; Latin name for garlic is Allium sativa, chromium picolinate, and niacin. Chromium is an essential mineral to balance insulin's regulation of carbohydrates, fats, and proteins. Chromium picolinate works with insulin to initiate thermogenesis, to reduce body fat and build lean muscle mass. Ionic minerals, the B vitamin Niacin, CoQ10, Devil's Claw, DHEA, Hawaiian Noni, Licorice, Psyllium fiber, Cholesterade, Ginko Biloba, Pau d' Arco, and Una de Gato improve glucose (sugar) control.

# XXII

# Digestion

---

I would like to take you back in time about four million years to understand how to achieve ideal health. Dr. Bryant Van of Texas A&M University studied prehistoric man's diet. The only way to do this was to analyze fecal material. He found primitive man ate primarily whole grains, vegetables, smaller amounts of fruits, nuts and seeds. Meat was rarely eaten, and only when they could catch some prey. We find the same basic diet over hundreds of thousands of years. Ten thousand years ago, man was still subsisting on grains, fruits and vegetables.

It wasn't until approximately two hundred years ago that large quantities of meat and dairy products entered our diet. There has been a reduction in the use of whole grains, fruits and vegetables since then and a continual increase in cholesterol intake. Within the last thirty years, unfortunately, there has also been an alarming increase in our diet of sugar, salt, fats, food additives and artificial foods. What are we going to see in the coming decades? What will be the health of our future generations? We need to understand the digestive system to grasp these problems.

The digestive process begins when you chew food and the salivary glands secrete saliva to help break down the food. It then goes down the gullet to the stomach where it encounters certain digestive enzymes. Next, it passes through the small intestine and is broken down further by digestive juices secreted by the pancreas, gallbladder and liver. The food goes down a long pathway in the small intestine, nearly 32 feet, where there is a tremendous absorption area. The little villi located here absorb much of the food, with the remainder moving to the large intestine and eventually passing out of the body.

When we talk about the food we eat, an analysis of packaged food labels of 10 years ago would show the term "crude fiber" was often used. This was an inaccurate measurement of the actual fiber content in food because they would boil the food in the presence of a weak acid or alkali. All that remained was cellulose and lignin and it was believed this was the amount of fiber in food. This was a critical mistake, though, because "dietary fiber," the term we now use, is truly the total amount of plant food remaining intact and undigested after passing through the small intestine. What we find remaining is not only cellulose and lignin, but also pentose, pectin, guar gums, bengal gram, etc. There are several different components to fiber itself.

Fiber acts like a sponge, retaining water as it passes through the small intestine. This is usually called roughage, which is a misnomer because it gives the impression the food you eat roughs up the intestinal tract. Instead, we should call it "softage," because as this undigested food passes through the lower digestive system, it acts like a sponge to absorb water and other fluids, creating large, soft stools that pass out of the body in a healthy manner.

If we ingest a radioactive isotope (enclosed in a tiny case), we can monitor its intestinal transient time (the amount of time it takes to pass through and out of the body). Generally, in a healthy individual it should pass out within 1 1/2 days. The shocking truth is for the average American, the transient time is over three days, and as long as two weeks in many elderly people! We then have the resultant health problems.

One problem that develops is the result of a large amount of intestinal pressure inside the abdomen, created as fiberless food passes through the digestive tract and pulls out all the fluid. As a result, you're left with little, hard, rock-like stools, which some people call "bullets" or "buttons". This problem is widespread because of the preponderance of animal products (meat, cheese, eggs, dairy products, etc.) in our diet. These foods are all totally digestible, and devoid of fiber. You need about two hundred grams (7 ounces) of intestinal content to reach the rectum and pass out of the body. If there is less than this amount, (the average American has only about 3 ounces) the body has to use all its pressure and muscles in the abdominal area to force these stools out of the body.

As a result, one of the problems, which will develop early on, is **hiatus hernia**, a condition in which the upper part of the stomach is pushed up through the diaphragm toward the thoracic area. This is the most common cause of heartburn because the gastric juices pool in this area and burn. We now know the hiatus hernia is clearly related to constipation. We also know hiatus hernia is not present in cultures, which follow a high fiber diet.

**Gallstones** can also develop from lack of fiber in the diet. The gallbladder, which contains bile salts and cholesterol, sprays these bile salts and substances over the food to help digestion. If there is a lack of dietary fiber, large concentrations of cholesterol develop in the gallbladder. Of course, we also develop high concentrations of cholesterol from eating high cholesterol foods and gallstones, usually, are made of cholesterol in crystallized form.

These stones can be dangerous because severe pain can result if they block off the little passageway from the gallbladder to the intestines. It's probably one of the most severe pains a person could ever experience, and is sometimes mistaken for appendicitis. The removal of the gallbladder is the most common operation in the U.S., approaching 500,000 yearly. The gallbladder is simply a collecting sack for bile from the liver. Removing the gallbladder does not solve the problem because stones can still form and lodge in the passageway between the liver to the intestines. This could lead to jaundice and some very serious side effects.

We have found if you increase fiber in the diet, while also decreasing cholesterol and fat intake, the following will happen:

1. The fiber, especially water-soluble fiber, removes cholesterol from the body and the intestines. This helps to keep the balance of cholesterol to bile salts equal.

2. Fiber pulls more bile salts out of the body, which means instead of returning to the liver, the liver cholesterol has to be converted into additional bile salts.

3. A large intake of wheat fiber or water-insoluble fibers found in all types of grain increases the production rate of a solvent called chenodeoxycholate, which helps to keep these gallstones dissolved.
   Most people do not realize that gallstones can be dissolved instead of resorting to surgery. We have found diet can dissolve these gallstones, especially if they're caught in the early stages. We know of several patient case reports where gallstones have successfully dissolved. If you have stones,

have your doctor monitor your progress with the appropriate ultrasound or X-ray tests. Give yourself time and follow the Healthy Aging Plan very closely.

Another common digestive disorder is appendicitis. The appendix located near the end of the large intestine, looks like a little finger. We find the appendix often becomes infected in young people. It's the most common emergency surgery done in this country. It occurs more commonly in young people because the appendix is much narrower at a younger age. As you get older, it enlarges somewhat. If a young person suffers from a viral infection, the lymph also swells up because there is more lymph tissue in the appendix. If you are eating a low-fiber diet, without natural whole foods, the fecal material becomes so hard it can be trapped in the appendix and possibly lead to a serious infection, which is the cause of most appendicitis cases.

When I was in my early 20's, I was rushed to the hospital with incredible pain. All I could think was "Whatever you have to do to get rid of this pain, do it!" They removed my appendix, which was severely infected, and later told me they had saved my life on the operating table. I wish I had known ahead of time I could have prevented this painful experience through a whole, natural diet. I don't think any of you would want to go through this surgery, either. We suggest, therefore, young people start the program right away. **Following a high fiber, "softage" diet, can prevent appendicitis.** Food will not be trapped in the appendix, and because there is no hard fecal material, there is no cause for infection. In Third World countries, appendicitis rarely, if ever occurs because of their diet.

Another digestive disorder, also resulting from a lack of fiber, is **diverticulosis.** This disease affects one out of every three adults past the age of sixty, and one out of ten younger people. It occurs when the intestinal tract begins to form bursts or bubbles along the way. **Constipation** leads to high pressure inside the intestine that form bubbles along the walls called diverticuli. Although this doesn't always lead to serious side effects, sometimes it can become infected and then you have a problem called diverticulitis. But, this also can be avoided by increasing natural fibers in the diet.

Research studies now show when you increase the fiber, it reduces the pressure in the intestines, and often there is no need for surgery. This is an exciting development - to know we can avoid the serious consequences related to diverticulosis. Unfortunately, some doctors still recommend a low-fiber, bland diet for diverticulosis and this is a very dangerous mistake.

Over 50% of the American population suffer from **hemorrhoids**, or piles. We always hear jokes about hemorrhoids and commercials for hemorrhoid relief, but it's serious if you have them. The process leading to this condition begins at the soft, anal cushion near the end of the rectum that is there to retain the fecal material at appropriate times. But, if you build up pressure in the intestines from lack of fiber, the constant pressure leads to a swelling of the blood vessels in this anal cushion. When hard, fecal material (which should be soft) passes by, the shearing pressure pushes these enlarged blood vessels and anal cushion out to the external part of the body. This can lead to itching, infection and very serious cases requiring surgery. Fortunately, here again, we have found the increase in fiber in the diet can relieve this extra pressure, and sometimes avoid the need for surgery. "Preparation H" and other similar products do not get to the cause of the problem, as does dietary fiber.

**Ulcerative colitis** and **spastic colon** are also caused by a lack of fiber and worsened by allergies to dairy products or other foods. Try a high fiber diet centered around the least allergy producing foods like whole grain brown rice, yams, squash and cooked noncitrus fruits. Then, each week add back in other grains, vegetables and fruits to identify foods that cause you digestive upset.

**Varicose veins** are another problem caused by a low-fiber diet. Over 50% of men and women past the age of fifty have these unsightly veins throughout their legs. Usually they occur in the blood vessels in the leg are located very near the skin, and are not surrounded by muscle to help maintain support. When pressure is built up in the intestines from constipation and straining to evacuate hard fecal material, the blood in the veins gets pushed back. This pressure damages the valves that are designed to allow blood to flow up toward the heart again; if these one-way valves get pushed backward, all the blood pools in the veins, causing them to distend and become swollen and very unsightly.

The high fiber, natural foods help to prevent the formation of varicose veins. But, once they do form, it is questionable whether they can be reduced because of the severe valve damage in the vein. In that case surgery is usually done or they tie off the flow of that vein. Varicose veins are preventable, and if they have already developed, the Healthy Aging Plan can prevent further occurrence and development of these unsightly veins.

It should be noted varicose veins are not present in other cultures. Many people believe varicose veins are caused by pregnancy, but in cultures where the women give birth to as many as nine children, such as the Bantus of Africa, varicose veins don't occur. The Bantus eat a high fiber, natural diet that prevents this pressure build-up. Some people have suggested standing on your feet all day cause varicose veins. Barbers, who stand all day, were compared to other groups who don't stand regularly, and no greater incidence of varicose veins was found. Of course, standing may irritate the situation somewhat, but a high fiber diet makes a difference in our digestive tract.

If you are having problems passing a large, soft stool at least once or more each day, or if they are hard, rock-like stools; begin adding at least one heaping tablespoon of wheat bran to your daily diet. Sprinkle it in your whole grain cereal or soup, and within one week you should see improvement. If there is no improvement, then add another tablespoon after the first week; by the end of the third week you may have to add another. Keep adding fiber in this fashion until you find how much is needed to maintain regularity.

Many people believe they eat a high fiber diet because they eat salads. Salads are very high in water content and low in fiber. The best source of fiber is wheat bran, which is very concentrated. Buy the coarse type of Miller's wheat bran, which does the job much better than the fine type of bran. The second best sources would be the whole grains: brown rice, millet, corn, rye, etc. Next would be the legumes group, including beans, peas, nuts and seeds. Root vegetables such as carrots, potatoes and parsnips are the fourth best sources of fiber. The fifth and least sources of dietary fiber would be fruits and vegetables (unless you're large 48 oz. Servings twice a day). Man was meant to eat a high fiber, natural diet for good health. Avoid foods without fiber like meat and dairy products.

**Supplements** for good digestion include milk-free Lactobacillus Acidophilus, Alfalfa, Aloe Vera, Cascara Sagrada, Cayenne (Capsicum), Digestive Enzymes, Thyme, Golden Seal, Hawaiian Noni, Hawthorn Berry, Myrrh, Garlic, Pau d' Arco, Una de Gato, Papaya tea, Psyllium Fiber and Wild Yam.

# XXIII

# Healthy Aging Wellness Plan for Companies

The Healthy Aging Wellness Program can save a company a lot of money and greatly increase the productivity of employees just by promoting fitness, nutrition and healthier lifestyles among the workers. Here are some of the startling statistics to illustrate part of the problem:

Medical care accounts for a large portion (over 60%) of the total cost of workers' compensation.
- Industry pays out nearly $10 billion each year for sick pay.
- Total annual cost of health care in the U.S. now exceeds $225 billion, which equals about 9 percent of the Gross National Product---and that figure escalates every year.
- One hundred thousand worker deaths each year are caused by cardiovascular disease.
- Seven hundred million dollars are spent annually by business to replace workers who are out sick.

The burden to business and consumers alike of the astronomical cost of employee health care is illustrated rather dramatically by still another example: Except for wages, the highest single monetary component of the cost of a new General Motors automobile is the cost for its employees' health insurance premiums. They paid more for health insurance premiums than it has paid for purchasing steel to go into the automobiles! Realizing that bad health on the job is getting out of hand, many American executives are taking a cue from abroad in ways to solve their problems.

For example, the Japanese have long recognized the joys of fitness and of well-balanced health on the job. Their diet is centered on rice, vegetables and low-fat soy products. Their employees regularly

257

participate in "exercise breaks" rather than in the traditional American style coffee break. Upon coming to work first thing in the morning, Japanese workers gather together for stretching and light calisthenics, and then they go up to their desks or work places to start their day fresh and alert. Another exercise session in the middle of the afternoon gives them the energy to get through the afternoon doldrums that so often lull American workers into lethargy and make them look forward to 5 o'clock more than to the tasks at hand.

In visiting with several corporations, including Yamaha Motor Company. It was most impressive to observe the employer' employee relationship and to visit one of their rest and conditioning centers in Sendai, Japan. Employees and families are encouraged to use these facilities, and certainly, they are first-class! With such personal attention to their needs, it is easy to see why an employee feels so loyal about his or her company and why Japanese productivity is the highest in the world.

And the Japanese are not the only foreign nation to see the benefits of fitness. Workers in the Soviet Union have mandatory exercise sessions at their work places. So you can see the value of an alert, healthy worker hasn't been lost on the Soviet Government.

Some American companies have seen that part of the answer to their productivity and absenteeism problems may lie in the experience of the Japanese and Russians in promoting exercise. The result has been an increase in the number of American businesses that have started aerobic fitness programs, which are often called "wellness" programs. However, they do not encompass all of the essential components.

Wellness programs, which are being, implemented in both the hospital environment and in industry, must consist of much more than just initiating an exercise program. They must concentrate on at least five things:

1. Proper weight, diet, nutrition and supplementation.
2. Properly implemented and supervised exercise programs.
3. Reduction and/or elimination of cigarette smoking.
4. Prevention and rehabilitation of alcoholism or drug abuse.
5. Assessment of values and goals with stress and time management.

Corporations have found success in implementing one or more of these programs, and the employee response to them has been quite positive.

Generally speaking, an American wellness program is designed both to perk up employees during work hours and also to increase their overall employee attitudes and morale at work. It should screen employees for potential risks with recommendations for improving a person's coronary risk profile with diet and exercise suggestions.

Here are some encouraging signs, which may make companies want to try to start a similar program.

Between 1979 and 1982 business invested nearly $2 billion to establish and maintain wellness programs. But they don't have to be super sophisticated to work. All that's really required is good employer leadership to motivate the employees to use the exercise facilities regularly and the addition of healthy cafeteria foods, salad bars, with low-fat dressing, fruit, and blender vegetable drinks. Self-insured payors and providers have been able to reduce their expenditures by 40% by encouraging wellness and fitness programs.

Doctors who scoff at the value of preventive medicine in reducing employee absences-and there are still far too many of these medical skeptics-haven't talked to the Canadian Life Assurance Company, whose results have been particularly impressive. After a fitness program was started at the company, employee absentee rates were cut by 43 percent, and the savings to the company were $175,000 in 1 year. Also, employee turnover dropped by 13.5 percent, with savings estimate at $510,000.

Another large insurance company, Prudential, also needs no convincing about the benefits of wellness programs. After starting their program, they reported sharp declines in absenteeism (down over 50%), with estimate savings to the company in 1 year of $284,744.

Kennecott Copper showed a 55 percent decrease in medical costs, a saving they attributed to their wellness program. Their workers compensation was reduced by almost one half a million dollars!

New York Telephone carefully analyzed the results of its health promotion program to see exactly how much money they were saving in employee absences and in cost of medical treatment. Smoking cessation programs were credited with savings of $645,000. Also, reduction in cholesterol levels saved them $250,000 in medical costs, and hypertension control programs meant another $663,000 in savings.

Some companies also manage to save money through refunds on health insurance premiums. For example, Bonnie Bell Cosmetics, which has for years been promoting exercise and fitness among its employees, reported that for two consecutive years, their health insurance carrier gave the company a $43,000 refund on their premiums. The reason for this is that as the claims against insures decreased within their company, the cost of carrying the insurance became less-and so the savings were passed on to the company.

Another refund success story involves Forney Engineering in Dallas. This company instituted a wide-ranging wellness program, which encourages exercise, proper diet, and control of cigarette smoking. Because of their dramatically improved record of health claims, their insurance carrier recently gave them a $92,000 refund on their premium inpatient hospital stay insurance.

In an interesting twist on motivating employees to participate in these wellness programs, Bob Schwartz of the Schwartz Meat Company in Norman, Oklahoma, started an aerobics program among his 75 employees several years ago. He offered bonuses to workers who earned a minimum number of points from using the program every week for 6 months. At the end of the 6 months, the employee received an additional week's pay if he or she had participated, one-half week's pay was added. If an employee, his or her spouse, and two children faithfully participated in the program for 1 year, at the end of that time there would be a 1-½ month salary bonus. Is such a program realistic?

This answer is a resounding "yes!" The results of this incentive program were dramatic, with productivity shooting up and absenteeism dropping sharply. And perhaps the best indication of employee morale came from the employees themselves. While many other companies are having labor battles, Bob Schwart's employees saved up enough money out of their own pockets to send him and his wife to Europe for 4 weeks-all expenses paid!

So there is a great deal to be said for wellness programs in corporations from everyone's point of view, boss and employee alike. If your company doesn't have such a program, you may be able to help organize one. Here are some points based on suggestions by Blue Cross/Blue Shield to help you along:

- Talk to people in companies that have programs. Find out how much their approach to fitness costs and whether or not they would change anything they've set up.
- Organize a committee, draft a wellness program proposal, and set a deadline within which you want to accomplish your goals.
- Take advantage of in-house expertise of company doctors and employees trained in fitness-related fields and nutrition.
- Publicize your idea to gain support among the employees in the company.
- Include employees' families in the program: Remember that they too, are on your company health plan.
- Get top executives committee to the program since they will be the ones who will have the greatest influence in getting the idea approved.
- Evaluate and change your wellness program periodically to suit your evolving needs.
- Use community resources whenever possible. Local schools and gyms may be able to help provide facilities and instruction, thus reducing your costs.

Many corporations are hiring their own staffs and building their own facilities, but that may be an unnecessary luxury. IBM started a national program for its employee that has been highly successful without involving an expensive building program. Instead of erecting facilities or paying for memberships in various clubs, contractual arrangements are made with local groups to provide educational and training programs for employees and families.

For example, if ten or more employees and family members want a 5-day, quit smoking program, IBM will make all the arrangements and pay the bill. Likewise, if there is interest in an aerobic dance class, IBM will contract with an instructor, make arrangements for a place, and pay the bill. Direct contractual arrangements with YMCAs, driver education courses, and weight-loss programs have all been highly successful. It is a new approach to employee wellness programs that is enjoying great popularity among IBM personnel.

But even though the business community is beginning to come around to the idea that participants in wellness programs reap many corporate rewards, the biggest changes yet to be made will focus on the life and health insures. Some life insurance companies already offer discounts on premiums to people who do well on a physical exam, exercise regularly, and don't smoke. Why the premium breaks? It's simply that those who take care of their health have a lower risk of early death.

However, health insurers so far don't offer the same incentives. Even if you watch your weight and diet, don't smoke, and exercise regularly, you still pay the same premium as the person who isn't as conscientious. Over the last three years Managed Care Organizations has started providing additional preventative services. It has been found that for every dollar spent on preventative medicine, ten to twenty dollars are saved on care. Managed care organizations insures have been encouraged to get more involved in good health programs.

An old Chinese custom was for the people to pay their physician only when they were well. If they got sick, the doctor had to care for the patient without any pay. That was quite an incentive for doctors to work hard at keeping people well! With the increasing baby boomer population needing care and the payment methodologies that are more prevalent with managed care; physicians must change the way in which they practice medicine. Motivation to educate patients and reduce the number of physician office visits is essential.

So you can see that establishing a personal balance that will lead to total well being on the job is not limited to one individual's commitment to fitness. If we hope to create an environment where good health and productivity become the order of the day, we must all work together- to achieve community equilibrium, based on good nutrition and aerobic conditioning, which will accrue to the benefit of all.

# XXIV

∞

# Summary of Results

---

The following is a report of 643 people that were tested for cholesterol, triglycerides, blood morphology, carotid artery scan, weight, and blood pressure. The study began in the San Diego area of La Jolla, California with the Tony Robbins Mastery program participants. On March 19-20, 1992 participants were tested for starting lipid levels and vital statistics listed above. The same participants were re-tested nine days later March 28 and 29, 1992 after they all had been provided daily low-fat, water –rich, complex carbohydrate meals, without animal products. Several guest speakers including **Dr. Nick Delgado** and Tony Robbins provided **education** and **motivational** seminars. Exercise was daily **walking**, or **jogging** for 30 minutes to one hour. Also, **Dancing** followed by group **massage** sessions lasting approximately ten minutes was conducted nearly four times a day, during the seminar breaks.

Another group of participants with a similar regime of diet, exercise, education and motivation lectures were tested at Mastery University in Hawaii on August 20-22, 1992 and re-tested nine days later on August 29 and 30, 1992 after following the wellness program. The results of the total 643 people tested at the start of Mastery University and re-tested within 7 to 9 days upon the completion were summarized as follows.

The data showed a dramatic reduction in triglyceride averaging over 33% reduction in those with elevated levels over 150 mg/dl even after meals! The drop in total cholesterol in those with elevated levels over 180 was over 25% within nine days. Over half the group was able to achieve ideal levels for lipids and sustain these levels. By changing behaviors, examining values, setting goals, and taking immediate action this program is one of the most successful, life changing programs of it's type in the country. I continued to test and lecture at Mastery University with Tony Robbins from 1992 until 1997. Now, I am setting up wellness programs for hospitals and medical groups.

Triglycerides over 151 to 500 reduced by 42% in 9 days in 126 people
Triglycerides of 101 to 150 reduced by 24% in 9 days in 182 people
Triglycerides less than 199 mg/dl remained in safe range in 335 people. Repeat tests six months later showed continued compliance and maintenance.

Dramatic cholesterol reductions were seen in those with the highest initial levels. Follow-up at one year showed excellent results. The "Bad" Cholesterol LDL dropped the most, and HDL the "good" cholesterol ratio improving toward a 1 to 3 ratio or better.

Cholesterol over 200 reduced by 30% in 9 days in 136 people
Cholesterol of 160 to 199 reduced by 21% in 9 days in 226 people
Cholesterol of 100 to 159 reduced by 6% in 9 days in 291 people

This data reports the statistically significant drop in both cholesterol and triglycerides levels. Microscopes connected to TV monitors were used to demonstrate improvements in circulation and separation of red blood cells as fat was reduced after only nine days. Carotid artery screenings was used to education and warn those with atherosclerosis to comply with the suggested dietary changes. Blood pressure dropped to ideal levels in over 85% of those with initial elevated levels. This compared favorable to other wellness programs I've worked with such as the Pritikin Plan.

Over half of the group was re-tested six months to a year later, with an estimated 80% compliance to the diet and exercise. This remarkable compliance to the Healthy Aging type plan was confirmed by a two weekly food and exercise recall record taken on each participant. Continued improvements in fat loss, lipid reductions, cardiac risk ratio and blood pressure normalization was measured six months later. Body fat reduced noticeably within six months without starvation.

Matched control groups with people tested for pre-employment blood pressure, lipid and body fat testing at companies without nutrition and wellness programs, had no significant drop in cholesterol (less than 10% reduction), triglyceride, body fat, or blood pressure.

The following is an example of sample menus served to all the participants and an activity schedule:

Sunday August 23, 1992
7:30 to 8am: **Exercise** starts with walking or running using a heart monitor at 180 minus the persons age x .65 for the target heart exercise level.

8 to 8:30am: **Breakfast** - Fruit (mangos, strawberries, honeydew melon, pineapple), muffins (with some sugar and oil prepared by the hotel).

9 to 10am: **Lectures,** 10 to 10:20 am: **Dance and Massage** (high intensity music: Contemporary rock and roll).

10:20am to 1:00pm: **Lectures,** 1:00pm to 1:15pm: **Dance**
1:15pm to 2:30 p.m.: **Lectures**

2:30pm: **Lunch** - raw salad of carrots, bean sprouts, cucumbers, romaine lettuce, and iceberg lettuce, dressing of either Caesar or Italian (8 grams of fat per tablespoon). Also the participants were served a casserole of sliced potatoes, mixed with corn and enchilada sauce and a wheat roll.

3:00pm to 6pm **Lectures, Dance** 6-6:15pm, **Lectures** 6pm to midnight

The menus varied each day, yet similar to the above examples. Low-fat vegetarian foods have a quick digestion time with natural enzymes, and regular exercise makes it necessary to nibble or snack frequently on fresh fruits, veggies, and bread nearly every hour or two. Many participants who did not nibble or snack, reported feeling very hungry or weak at times. About fifty of the participants used the cool tote to carry a supply of fresh foods to nibble between the three meals. Several of those people who nibbled properly (whenever they felt weak or slightly hungry they would eat a small amount of fresh food) reported a consistent feeling of well being and energy.

The intervention of exercise helps to reduce triglycerides, however cholesterol reduction was accomplished primarily by the Healthy Aging diet. Other studies have shown that exercise by itself does not lower cholesterol levels significantly. The zero cholesterol diet would account for the 20 to 30% drops in cholesterol in those people with initial elevated levels.

The 20 to 40% drop in triglycerides would result from the combination of diet and exercise. The fat content of diet used in this study averaged less the 30 grams of fat per day. Participants had buffet selections including the availability of fatty salad dressings and butter. However, the overall diet was less than 15% calories coming from fat, 10 to 15% protein (all vegetable protein in origin) and 70 to 80% complex carbohydrates and about 5% to 10% simple carbohydrates with zero to 10 mg. of cholesterol per person per day.

In the future, we would suggest a low-fat alternative such as apple butter, butter buds, and a nonfat salad dressing or salsa will contribute what we believe to be even better results. If the initial triglycerides were low to begin with, a slight rise could occur (but usually within an acceptable range). Some of the elevated triglyceride levels occurred most likely because of the excessive use of fruit juice (4 to 6 glasses in a day) by some participants. Those people, who ate whole fruit, while using less than a glass of fruit juice a day, did not show a rise in triglycerides.

The Healthy Aging diet of fruits, vegetables, grains, beans, peas, nuts, seeds, under 10% fat, 12% protein, over 70% Complex carbohydrates meals is essentially cholesterol free (less than 5 mg day)...No animal product, No dairy, little or no added oils. Daily exercise, dance, walking, jogging per pulse monitor target improved results.

The data for cholesterol and triglycerides were provided by twelve Reflotron testing units from Boehringer Mannheim, calibrated with code strips, tested against known values and collected by trained medical assistants. Cholestech units were used for lipid panels in future studies we conducted. The weight scales were balanced physician scales. The Morphology test was done on Ziess microscopes and phase contrast lens, with a Panasonic video camera and Sony TV for viewing by the participants. A Diasonic DRF10, Hewlett Packard, and Johnson & Johnson provided carotid artery imaging with a photograph from a Sony printer for each participant to detect early signs of atherosclerosis. Blood pressures were taken with standard cuffs and stethoscopes.

Virtually every participant reported increased energy, a sense of well being and determination to continue to follow the new healthy lifestyle of diet, exercise and managing mental states. In 1998 I visited a major hospital in-patient and out patient program in Chicago. Their program included a well-designed exercise training session offered at least three times a week and lasting from one to six months. Dietary training offered by a staff dietician that was only provided upon request or if a patient had extremely elevated lipid levels. Records show a need for a more intensive weekly inpatient and outpatient education programs for nutrition, lipid management and lifestyle re-education.

## The **HEALTHY AGING PLAN** for **Wellness & Therapy**

1. **Blended drinks** consuming at least one serving (48 oz each) a day of - sprouts, veggies, and fruit. Large **salads** (with nonfat dressings) at least once or twice a day. Consume at least 80% of your diet from raw food, 20% cooked food- Brown rice or basmati rice and other complex carbohydrates. Avoid all fat and cholesterol foods meats, dairy, eggs, oil.

2. **SUPPLEMENTS**:

**Hormone balance**: (if tested deficient on saliva, urine & blood) added progesterone cream daily, melatonin (sublingual), DHEA(spray or liposome cream), homeopathic human growth factor IGF-1 and Human growth hormone, secretagogues from soy protein isolate, GABA, Suma (Brazilian Ginseng), Damiana, straw oats (Avena Sativa) and Saw Palmetto.

**Digestive Enzymes**-in capsules (Amylase, Protease, Lipase, Cellulase) consumed with cooked food.

**Herbs**- Aged Garlic Extract (allium sativa), Ginkgo Biloba, Native legend tea, Una de Gato, Barley greens, chlorophyll, Bayberry, catnip, chickweed, fenugreek, getian, golden seal, irish moss, myrrh, blue vervain, comfrey, St. John's Wort, yellow dock, cyani, mandrake, fennel, Milk thistle, grapefruit, pectin and acerola, echinacea, burdock, dandelion, cayenne.

**Phytochemicals**- PhytoGen ( soy phytochemicals rich in genistein), Phyto Veggie & fruit capsules, Indoles (cruciferous vegetables) Bioflavonoids, Fructooligosaccharide (cellulose, legume apple pectin).

**Antioxidants**- Grape seed (OPC), Peruvian cat's claw,(Uncaria Tomentosa)

**Minerals**- ionic 92 elements, calcium, magnesium, zinc, selenium, potassium

**Vitamins**- Multi-vitamin formulas derived from whole food complexes A, E, C, B-complex, B-12

**Essential fatty acids**- Evening primrose & flax seed

**Shark cartilage extract-Glucosamine**

**Fiber**- Cholesterade (Gum Arabic), Oat bran, Metamucil (pysllum).

3. **Far-Infrared-Wave** & **Magnets** (sports wraps, seat pads, comforter).
4. **Exercise** & daily walks 30 minutes or more per session
4. Be resourceful **positive state of mind-** ask power questions, enjoy comedy, funny movies, supportive friends, pray and attend to your spiritual life.

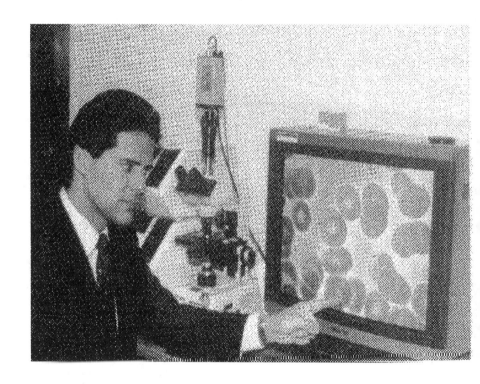

# XXV

# International Health Dynamics Wellness Program For Hospitals & Physicians

Modern health care is designed to be focused on illness. As of January 1999 federal law will mandate hospital and Managed Care Organization wellness program implementation. Presently, less than 60% of hospitals and physician groups are providing the critical active education and nutrition programs to patients and members. The cover story in Newsweek (March 98) points out that rather than contribute to bypass surgery's annual $26 billion price tag, more than forty major insurance companies now cover wellness alternatives, and Medicare is soon to follow.

Prompting a revolution in American medicine, International Health Dynamics realizes the importance of taking an aggressive pro-active approach to prevention as well as the cure of disease, and has been focused on this goal with the public as well as private industry for over twenty years. Wellness impacts a patients entire life and equates to much more that simply "not being ill" - incorporating positive lifestyle changes of health and well being. Through education the patient is encouraged to consider all aspects of their environment as we focus on the personal responsibility of maximum health.

Achieving wellness can be difficult, especially when major lifestyle changes are necessary for the patient to have the optimum outcome long term. What clearly sets us apart is our unique yet simple approach to education through fluid systems and presentations that are integrated in the spirit of fun, laughter, comedy and music that facilitates easy learning that is entertaining and enjoyable for all ages.

Exceptional results in on-going hospital studies have spurred on an overwhelming acceptance of International Health Dynamics Health and Wellness Programs. An increasing number of patients have successfully overcome life-threatening diseases like heart disease, prostate tumors, diabetes, and hypertension by turning the clock back by using this proactive approach. Each program has been carefully designed to address the special concerns common to the specific diagnosis, and for those who desire to make lifestyle changes. Our programs are customized to meet specific needs and challenges of hospital and physician care plans. Our Health and Wellness Program continues to be embraced by the mainstream in medicine.

One of our main goals is instilling in the patient the need for new commitment to wellness and to understand the degrees of wellness. Wellness education should begin at any point of patient care. Our focus is assisting patients to move, as far towards optimum health, therefore experiencing the best life has to offer. Even within a short hospital stay (two to nine days) substantial changes in blood and urine chemistries have been observed and documented.

A healthy diet doesn't have to be boring, dull, and tasteless! A large array of options and alternatives of diet as well as technologically superior supplementation keep patients looking forward to sampling the many different meals that are high water content, high fiber and nutrient rich. Diet is one of the most important aspects of a change for a more healthy future. Teaching the patient how to improve their diets and begin a conditioning program that will work for them is critical. The principles of wellness learned through International Health Dynamics Wellness Program will set the stage for the family's future of sound nutrition. We stress follow-up programs that involved both the patients and their families to ensure the **highest rate of patient compliance**. Where it becomes essential that other family members are in need of recovery or wellness program education, we offer a specific program that included individual counseling, group education, lectures, multi-media, and other types of assistance and encouragement.

What is the future of health worth? Regardless of the mandate taking effect in January 1999, an educated health conscious individual is an asset to any company, hospital and to the nation.

## GOALS of the Education System

PRIMARY GOAL: The goal is to provide the highest cost effective primary and secondary health care solutions through exceptional services to the patients, family and community in an environment of education, teaching and action.

**Acute Patient**: The goal is to initially stabilize and then reverse the clinical symptoms associated with the diagnosis with an emphasis on education. This will reduce hospital stay, return symptoms of disease, and improve the overall patients' care received. First and second hand nursing personnel, ancillary departments such as dietary, physical therapy, and physical therapy efforts will all be centered around the patients' necessary educational needs. We are providing group and individual education sessions with the patients to meet the patients needs and questions more efficiently.

**Non-Acute Patient**: The need here is to help patients to stabilize symptoms associated with the diagnosis of degenerative disease. We will reduce future hospital visits and lengths of stay, because of a reduction and prevention of recurrent symptoms, subsequent diagnosis or complicating conditions.

**Outpatient**: The goal is to educate patients and the assisting family as to the necessary lifestyle modifications in nutrition, exercise and the reduction in risk factors associated with degenerative diseases and diagnosis that may exacerbate and require additional health care needs. We want to establish our wellness ideal model in each patient's daily life and to instill a permanent lifestyle change.

## Measurable Outcome for the Learner

To be able to identify and implement increased frequency of exercise, improvement in dietary selection both at home and dining out to thoroughly understand and concept of ideal blood lipids and chemistries. The following goals will be realized within the first four days and then re-evaluated at two and four week intervals. Thereafter, monthly evaluations need to made, until complete remission of or restoration of normalcy is achieved:

## 4-DAY GOALS

The average reduction in total lipids, cholesterol and LDL should be 20-30% of baseline entry levels, with ideal measurements as follows:

- Reduce LDL cholesterol to less than 95/mg/dl, with total cholesterol of less than 180 mg/dl. The cardiac risk factor of less than 3 to one HDL, LDL ratio. Reduction of VLDL of less than 40 mg/dl.
- Triglycerides, fasting level of less than 100 mg/dl and a 4-hour postprandial (after a low fat high fiber low sugar meal) will be less than 140 mg/dl. Fasting glucose levels will drop between 60-100 mg/dl and under 130 mg/dl, within four hours after a meal.
- With a nutritional protocol of frequent small meals ingested throughout the day and education for eating to anticipate hunger and avoiding gorging, we can expect 30% less serum insulin output and 20% less c-peptides output and a reduction in cortisol in the urine.
- A 10-15% reduction in blood pressure both systolic and diastolic measures. There will be concurrent needs to monitor and reduce blood pressure medication within the first 14-30 days as reductions occur. At least 60% of patients should be free of all types of hypertension medication at the end of a 30-day treatment and follow-up program.
- Symptoms of digestive disorders such as constipation or diarrhea will be both regulated and restored to normalcy because of the high dietary fiber content of the meal plan along with supplemental fiber added to the diet both soluble and insoluble.
- Reported improvement in symptoms such as fatigue, depression, with a reduction in platelet aggregation, and red blood cell clumping.

- Note: There may be a slight reduction in HDL cholesterol in the first week on the plan, however, because of the significant drop in LDL the cardiac risk ratio will conclude in favorable levels.

## Topics to be Covered in Education Wellness Program

How to maximize patient compliance with the interactive "tell, see, do" lifestyle and exercise wellness program.

Mass media application through weekly presentations on tape, television and or radio programming to be aired at convenient times and addressed in a format that encourages and interactive atmosphere and is consistent to the learners age, literacy level, primary language, and cultural lifestyle and beliefs. Video and audio education programs will be offered in the reception / education rooms in the Primary Care Physicians' office, as well as the designated hospital education rooms or cafeteria during mealtimes. The hospital or medical group's in-house coordinator will facilitate the distribution and compliance of patient education through these means.

Educational handbooks in English and Spanish covering most common diagnosis, their associated diagnosis and complications of care will be broken out into patient status and staff involvement. These will be provided for the education of the patient, the staff, and the physicians. Additional languages will be provided dependent on demographic need. With the proper budget, character coloring books and audiotapes to teach children a healthy and fun approach to good nutrition and exercise, is available. The patient's family will learn integration of health with other values of love, security and relationships.

- Computer programming within all facilities to be set up to ensure compliance in all areas - to facilitate a stopgap for physician and staff compliance as well. To be utilized to gather and monitor statistics regarding the Wellness Program.

- We have available a CD-ROM wellness educational system, with this book and other hard copy literature. We plan to involve an interactive web site for the use of all patients, physicians and staff. Collection of personal data, progress, questions, and attendance information with follow up seminars or events will be forwarded to the medical chart as formal documentation of attendance and/or on-going participation. There are a Direct link-up with participating facilities regarding the forwarding of information on additional specific health education needs. By directly linking up patients with the appropriate department or hospital liaison, we can schedule and assist them. With their health problems. In this way we can identify each persons health education needs and refer each member to utilize the appropriate service. Some patients may be in need of prenatal classes, parenting classes, smoking cessation, or diabetes management, etc. Then we can address each person's questions, health status, family role or situation.

# Hospital Wellness Program

One of the largest problems with the delivery of health care is the lack of understanding by patients and clinicians about how to integrate education and wellness training into the care plans being provided. The resources to understand one another have been dispersed and separated throughout health care history. Now we are seeing an increase demand due to managed care and other payor contracts that both patients and physicians must learn the business of wellness rather than just treating diseases.

In association with International Health Dynamics, we have an opportunity to assist hospitals and primary care physicians groups in developing the Healthy Aging and Wellness plan. This partnership helps bridge the gap between the clinician and patients and is designed to meet the needs of all patients being admitted to the hospital. The out patient follow-up programs are also designed and enhanced to help hospital staff members and physicians to benefit.

The combined efforts of hospitals, physicians and payors with the assistance of International Health Dynamics will become the most comprehensive and complete program to meet the demands of the industry. It is an accurate and easy to use program for empowering health care interests to develop a successful system.

This program includes step by step instructions to building an effective Wellness program for example a cafeteria style buffet for staff and patients would be included and is outlined in the coming section.

Phase I begins at the hospital, in-patient care, for newly admitted patients with any or all of the following diagnosis:
Peripheral Vascular Disease
Acute Myocardial Infarction
Cardiovascular Disease
Unstable Angina
Cancer
Diabetes
Hypertension

Stroke

Digestive Disorders, constipation, gallstones, ulcers

With this education and treatment wellness plan hospitals and facilities will save substantial amount of money by reducing return and recurring hospital stays for the same diagnosis and symptomatology.

Wellness Program Treatment/Education Guidelines will be integrated into nursing care plans and stronger inpatient and outpatient education programs. Specific programs have detailed education needs such as:

- Acute Patients: 9 days education training with 2 months follow-up
- Non-Acute Patients: 3-4 days training with 2 months follow-up
- Outpatient Patients: 2 -5 days training with 1 month follow-up

Current medical treatments will be modified to address specific preventative and educational requirements such as:

**Non-Ambulatory Patients**

Hospital staff must take proper aspiration precautions with acute patients, upon admission and swallow reflex must be tested prior to giving fluids. In conjunction with standard I.V treatments and protocol, the meals will follow the same menu plan of ambulatory patient, gradually being introduced to blended drink mixes as tolerated until complete whole food can be consumed. The patient will then be taken to meal buffet line and considered an ambulatory patient.

**Ambulatory Patient**

The patients will be directed to meal buffet line for between three and five meals a day (breakfast, snack, lunch, snack, dinner) and instructed by staff and educational literature (booklets) to go to the buffet area to eat, upon the first sign of hunger. Patients will learn to anticipate their hunger, identify their low energy levels, and eat as often as they feel weak or "empty". (This could potentially be three to eight meals a day for some patients). Frequent small meals will be encouraged, with overconsumption or gorging (i.e. one or two larger meals per day) discouraged and avoided completely.

**Food Composition:**

The composition of foods will be 10-15% fat, 10-15% protein (primarily vegetable-protein), and 70-80% water rich complex carbohydrates, with over 50% of the diet being raw and uncooked. Meals will be high in fiber, high water content, low fat, low in choleric density, utilizing vegetable food protein rather than animal protein, be dairy free with substantially decreased inclusion of wheat and flour products.

***Buffet style service implemented to promote patients taking a very active part in their own rehabilitation and wellness - learning lifestyle changes by fully integrating them in the systems and "educate through doing". Also served in an effort to reduce costs, because individual meals are not needed, so less time is required by a specialized dietary staff.

**Buffet-style meals to include:**
- Raw fruits and raw vegetables
- Blended drinks (between 32 and 64 oz. of blended raw vegetables choosing from a selection including carrots, broccoli, sugar snap peas, cucumbers, sugar beets, celery, apples with skin, watermelon, cantaloupe, honeydew melon, frozen pitted cherries, blueberries, strawberries, banana.) With a ratio of 2/3 vegetables & sprouts and 1/3 fruit.
- Raw salads (artichoke hearts, capers, palm hearts, tomatoes, red bell peppers, sugar snap peas, Chinese show peas, water chestnuts, broccoli, dark green lettuce, Napa cabbage, garbanzo beans, kidney beans, corn, peas, various sprouts) to include fat free dairy free salad dressings.
- Vegetable or minestrone soups
- Entree main course centered on brown rice, corn tortillas, legumes, potatoes, and salsa, Chinese, Italian, Mexican cuisine, etc.
- Condiments: Freshly made salsa and sauces, mustard, garlic and any spices to taste.

**Exclude from all diets fruit or vegetable juices that have been "juiced" opposed to being blended. All fiber content must remain intact.
**Progress to be monitored by a 1 hour and 4 hour blood testing on day one and day three.

**Supplementation to be administered both a.m. and p.m.**

An inclusion of a multi-vitamin (inclusive of B complex, B-12, anti-oxidant vitamins A-bet carotene, E, C, Essential fatty acids, ionic colloidal minerals, calcium, magnesium, iron, potassium, zinc, chromium picolinate, and other trace minerals) all derived from whole plant based origins in a delivery system preferably sublingual to maximize absorption and metabolic utilization. Capsule and tablet forms are also acceptable, with provisions for herbs and whole, organic sources.

**This program excluded all dairy-based whey protein powders/supplements.

Assessment of Biochemical Hormones & Natural Herbal Hormone Replacements:
The following tests would be optional but highly recommended for optimum results with all programs. Laboratory tests emphasizing 24-hour urine to assess the steroid hormones including all three estrogens, progesterone, testosterone, and DHEA. Blood testing for lipids, chemistries and IGF-1 and saliva tests for outpatients will also be performed when indicated.

**Monitored by 24 hour Urine Testing:**
Free & Total Testosterone,
 Estrodial
• Progesterone
• DHEA & Cortisol

**Additional Suggested testing when indicated:**
• Thyroid panels with TSH
• Insulin like growth factor 1, human growth hormone
• Melatonin
• Pregnenolone

Replacement with natural and herbal hormones (see Fountain of Youth chapter), (testosterone, progesterone, estrogen, DHEA, Melatonin, Pregnenolone, thyroid, human growth hormone, human growth factors etc.)

**Exercise Protocol**
Day 1   Active and passive range of motion and initiation into the first stages of walking program to tolerance.

Day 2-4 Increased frequency and duration of exercise sessions to tolerance. By Day 4 a 15-30 minute exercise walking session at least 3-5 times per day should be tolerated and encouraged.

Activity and Safety - Aerobic exercise, encouraged or assisted by nursing, physical therapy, cardiac rehabilitation, and Cardiopulmonary rehabilitation. A simple plan of walking exercise to maximum tolerance of between six minutes and thirty minutes sessions of three to six times per day. The intensity will remain within safe target heart rate and the avoidance of excessive respiratory exertion. Additional cross training exercises may include mini trampolines, recumbent bicycles and treadmill.

This Book and CD's will educate all staff members. At least once per day, patients will be required to read the book, listen to audio tapes, and view educational video tapes in their rooms, or in a audio/video check out area. Educational videos or material will be playing during the buffet line eating times.

The discharge planning for out patients will include the normal protocol and frequency of visits, however we suggest the addition of lipid & glucose blood test screening done at appropriate intervals.

Please contact the administration of your local hospitals or care providers if you want to implement the Healthy Aging wellness program.

**FINAL ENCOURAGING WORDS**:
What will you be like five or ten years from now if you don't even try the healthy aging program? Can you afford to wait until it is almost too late? Can you see yourself looking and feeling better than you have in years? How will the *healthy aging plan* help career, relationships and feeling of wellbeing?

You do have a choice. You could choose to do nothing and continue to do what you have been doing. Will you be happy with the rate at which you are aging? Is it worth the risk of illness, pain of degeneration and loss of function? You could try the Healthy Aging program for just 9 days. You will begin to feel better and have more energy almost immediately. This I know, because I have worked with and set up wellness programs and tested thousands of people upon starting the program of diet, exercise, supplements, and mental attitude adjustments. Do they work so quickly? Yes! This is great because it will motivate you to continue on the program. And if you go off the program, what will happen? You'll experience the difference and want to get back on track immediately. This will allow you to benefit from this program for a lifetime, because it will become a way of life for you. If you are age 30 or older the more dramatic the results will be.

# Keynote Seminars, Workshops, Corporations, School Assemblies

Nick is considered one of the top seminar leaders in the country on health, wellness and peak performance. Call 1-800-631-0232 to have Nick come speak to your group or company. Here is what participants have to say about Nick Delgado and his life changing seminars:

*"Simply put, It was the best I've heard yet."* M. Midgeth

*"Excellent! Very credible and informative. He has taken my understanding to a whole new level! Thanks!"* L. Dixon, Toronto

*"Very informative and enjoyable and most important motivates you to do it!"* M. Johnson, Louisiana

*"I've heard many lectures on healthy but I must say of all the lectures I've heard this one by far gave me the most practical and usable information."* Audie Champion

*"Dr. Delgado was very, very impressive in his presentation. I've been in the field of nutrition for 7 years and he's the best I've seen. I'd like to thank him for his contribution to life!"* B. Lany, NY

*"Conveys the message of health and wellness in an exceptionally motivating manner. After listening to Dr. Delgado you know that his message is a must!!!"* Sylvia Blouin, Baton Rouge, LA

## BIBLIOGRAPHY

Anderson, James W., MD. *Diabetes - A practical new guide to healthy living*. New York, New York: Arco Publishing, Inc., 1981.

Bailey, Covert. *The Fit-or-Fat Target Diet*. Boston, Massachusetts: Houghton Mifflin Co. 1984.

Bennett, Cleaves, MD. *In 12 weeks control your high blood pressure without drugs*. Garden City, N.Y: Doubleday & Co., Inc., 1984.

Bronfen, Nan. *Nutrition for a Better Life*. Santa Barbara, California: Capra Press, 1980.

Burkitt, Denis, MD., F.R.C.S., F.R.S. *Eat right - to stay healthy and enjoy life more*. New York, New York: Arco Publishing, 1979.

Cherniske, Stephen, M.S., *The DHEA Breakthrough*, New York, New York, Ballantine Books, 1996

Cranton, Elmer, MD., *Resetting the Clock*, New York, New York, M. Evans and Company, Inc., 1996

Crenshaw Theresa L., MD., *The Alchemy of Love and Lust* New York, New York, Putman Sons, 1996

Cummings, Stephen, MD., Ullman, Dana, M.P.H., *Everybodies Guide to Homeopathic Medicines*, L.A., CA, Jeremy P. Tarcher, Inc., 1991

Dunne, Lavon J. *Nutrition Almanac*. New York, New York: McGraw Hill Publishing Co., 1990.

Fossel, Michael, Ph.D., MD., *Reverse Human Aging*, New York, New York, William Morrow Co. 1996.

Guyton, Arthur C., MD. *Textbook of Medical Physiology*. Philadelphia, Pennsylvania: Sanders Co. 1976.

Howell, Edward, Dr., *Enzyme Nutrition*, Wayne New Jersey, Avery Publishing, 1985

Janson, Michael, MD., *The Vitamin Revolution*, Greenville, New Hampshire, Arcadia Press, 1996

Klaper, Michael, MD. *Pregnancy, Children & Vegan Diet*. Umatilla, Florida:Gentle World Inc. 1987

Klatz, Ronald, Dr., *Grow Young with HGH*, New York, New York, Harper Collins, 1997

Wright, Klatz, Ronald, Dr., Goldman, Robert, Dr., *Stopping the Clock*, New Canaan, Connecticut, Keats Publishing, Inc., 1996.

Langley, Gill, MA, Ph.D. *Vegan Nutrition*. Oxford, England: The Vegan Society Ltd., 1988.

Leonard, Jon N., J.L. Hofer and Nathan Pritikin. *Live Longer Now* New York, New York, Charter 1974.

Ley, Beth, *DHEA Unlocking secrets to the Fountain of Youth*, Newport Beach, CA,BL Publications, 1996

Lovendale, Mark, *Quality Longevity*, Monarch Beach, CA, Advanced Health Care, 1998

Mayer, Bill, *Magic in Asking*, Solona Beach, CA, Bill Mayer, 1997

McDougall, John A., MD. *McDougall's Medicine*. Piscataway, New Y

**BIBLIOGRAPHY, cont.**

Jersey: New Century Pub, Inc., 1985.

McDougall, John A., MD., and Mary A. McDougall. *The McDougall Plan.* Piscataway, New Jersey: New Century Publishers, Inc., 1983.

Mindell, Earl, *Earl Mindell's Herb Bible*, New York, New York, Simon & Schuster, 1992

Neubauer, Richard, MD., Walker, Morton, DPM *Hyperbaric Oxygen Therapy*, Garden City Park, N. Y., Avery Publishing Group, 1998

Pritikin, Nathan. *Pritikin Permanent Weight Loss Manual.* New York, New York: Grosset Dunlap, 1981.

Pritikin, Nathan. *Pritikin Program Diet & Exercise.* New York, New York: Grosset Dunlap, 1979.

Ody, Penelope, *The Complete Medicinal Herbal*, New York, NewYork, Dorling Kindersley, 1993 Phillips, Nathaniel W. , *Anabolic Reference Guide*, Golden CO Mile High Publishing, 1991

Regelson, William, MD., Colman, Carol, *The Super Hormone Promise*, New York, N. Y, Simon & Schuster, 1996.

Robbins, John. *Diet for a New America.* Walpole, New Hampshire: Stillpoint Publishing, 1987.

Sattilaro, Anthony J., MD. *Recalled for Life.* New York, New York: Avon Books, 1982.

Shook, Edward, E. , Dr., *Advanced Treatise in Herbology*, Banning, CA, Enos Publishing Co., 1992

Swank, Roy Haver, MD., and Barbara Brewer Dugan. *The Multiple Sclerosis Diet Book.* New York, New York: Doubleday 1977

Webb, Denise, Ph.D., RD *The Complete "Lite" Foods Calorie, Fat Cholesterol Sodium Counter*, N.Y., New York: Bantam Books, 1990

Whitaker, Julian M., MD. *Reversing Diabetes.* New York, New York: Warner Books, Inc., 1987

Whitaker, Julian, MD. *Dr. Whitakers Guide to Natural Healing,* Rocklin, CA: Prima Press, 1995

Wieland, Bob, *One Step at a Time*, Grand Rapids, Michigan, Zonervan Books, 1989

Wright, Jonathan V., MD., Morgenthaler, John, *Natural Hormone Replacement*, Petaluma CA, Smart Publication, 1997

# INDEX

# To order additional copies of this book,

*Healthy Aging Breakthrough by Nick Delgado Ph.D.*, send a check or charge your credit card for $15.95 plus $3 shipping. How many copies would you like? ____

Name_____

Address_____

Phone:(AreaCode)Work_____Home_____

Credit Card (MC, Visa, American Express):

_____

Expiration Date_____

Signature:_____

Name of Product _____

**Send orders to:**
Nick Delgado
25422 Trabuco Rd. #105-141
Lake Forest, CA  92630

**Or call to place your order at 1-888-517-7421
or call for information at 1-800-631-0232**

# How to Look Great, Feel Younger and Stronger in 60 days

## Additional Products

### How to Look Great & Feel Sexy Cookbook    $15

This 400 page cookbook, "How to Look Great & Feel Sexy!" gives you the latest steps and recipes on nutrition to absorb vitamins, minerals, and hormones. You will learn techniques for achieving optimal mental attitude to achieve maximum health! Enjoy 600 tasty recipes: Italian, Chinese, Mexican, Thai, and American cusines.

### Health & Wealth Radio & TV Series 6 Cassette Tapes  $69

You will her the essence of the best interviews conducted by Dr. Nick Delgado on his radio and television programs. Discussions cover slowing the aging process using nutrition, natural hormones, herbs, exercise, stress reduction and smoking cessation. Tapes on humor, happiness, fitness, discipline for busy people, preserving the earth's resources, senile brain damage from meat, male sexual impotency, and the reversal of atherosclerosis.  Learn of relief for neck & back pain, improving circulation, skin rejuvenation, oxygen therapy, cosmetic procedures, supplements, homeopathy and allergies.

### Look & Feel Great 4 audio Tapes $49

The Look & Feel Great tapes explain how to establish new winning habits, lose unwanted body fat, and gain lean muscle tissue.  This program will bring you high-energy living.  Discover how to reduce cholesterol, triglycerides, and achieve ideal body weight.  Shop at the supermarket and order healthfully while dining out at almost any restaurant.

### Reverse Aging 4 audio tapes $49

The Reverse aging tapes teach how to replace biochemical hormones to slow aging. Also find out the cause and prevention of heart disease, diabetes, arthritis, cancer, osteoporosis, hypertension, hearing loss, digestive problems, ulcers, hernia, gallstones, and varicose veins.

### Wellness Video    $23.95

Nick's dynamic video tape of his most popular nutrition presentation will stimulate and motivate you to stay on the health track.  Filled with information that you can see and use now.